A GUIDE TO CARDIAC PACEMAKERS:
Supplement 1986-1987

A GUIDE TO CARDIAC PACEMAKERS:
Supplement 1986-1987

DRYDEN MORSE, M.D.

Clinical Associate Professor of Thoracic Surgery
Rutgers Medical School
New Brunswick, New Jersey
Director, Pacemaker Clinic
Deborah Heart and Lung Center
Browns Mills, New Jersey

ROBERT M. STEINER, M.D.

Professor of Radiology
Associate Professor of Medicine
Chief, Thoracic Radiology
Thomas Jefferson University School of Medicine
Philadelphia, Pennsylvania

VICTOR PARSONNET, M.D.

Director of Surgery
Director of the Pacemaker Clinic and the Pacemaker Foundation
Newark Beth Israel Medical Center
Newark, New Jersey

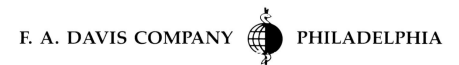

F. A. DAVIS COMPANY • PHILADELPHIA

Library of Congress Cataloging-in-Publication Data
Morse, Dryden P. (Dryden Phelps), 1924–
    A guide to cardiac pacemakers. Supplement, 1986–1987.

    Includes index.
    1. Pacemaker, Artificial (Heart)   2. Pacemaker, Artificial (Heart)—
Catalogs.   I. Steiner, Robert M.
II. Parsonnet, Victor, 1924–   III. Title.
[DNLM: 1. Pacemaker, Artificial.   WG 26 M884g 1983 Suppl. 1986–
87.
RC684.P3M665   1983   Suppl.   617′.412′0028   85–31126
ISBN 0–8036–6326–9

PREFACE

Since the publication of *A Guide to Cardiac Pacemakers,* in October 1983, progress in pacemaker technology has continued. Refinements in programming allow the physicians better choices of all pacemaker parameters. A startling increase in telemetry options, for example, has resulted in the ability to program into the pacemaker information concerning the patient's preoperative rhythm disturbances, and the date of implantation, and allows for pacemaker output measurement (in terms of pulse width and voltage). A list of all programmed parameters, and the date of the most recent programming together with telemetric display of intracardiac electrograms, a "marker" channel to identify when the pacemaker is actually sensing, and when it is firing in each cardiac chamber are available in some parameters. Many pacers will report on whether tachycardia (above the programmed upper rate limit) has occurred since the last programming.

Just which of the new pacemakers have some or all of these features is the subject of this supplement. Those pacemakers manufactured since 1983 by the leading companies in the United States are featured. Naturally, not every model of every manufacturer can be included.

Even as the volume goes to press, however, still newer pacemakers are on the drawing boards and in the planning stages by many companies. Because of the length of time it takes to publish books, it always happens that the very newest models are not included. This book, however, is primarily intended as a guide to the cardiac pacemakers that are already in patients in some quantities, and is intended to help physicians in identifying them. Consequently, new pacemakers for which x-rays and photographs are not available or which have arrived on the scene after the initiation of the publication process are not illustrated in this book.

Photographs and specifications of a representative group of programmers, pacing system analyzers, and monitors are also supplied.

A Guide to Cardiac Pacemakers: Supplement 1986–1987 is meant to be used with the previous book (also published by F. A. Davis), which includes pacemakers manufactured in the decade before 1983.

The authors particularly wish to thank the manufacturers for their cooperation in furnishing the authors with photographs, x-rays, and specifications of their various models.

Dryden Morse, M.D.
Robert M. Steiner, M.D.
Victor Parsonnet, M.D.

CONTRIBUTORS

ALAN D. BERNSTEIN, Eng.Sc.D.

Director of Technical Research, Department of Surgery
Technical Director, Pacemaker Center
Newark Beth Israel Medical Center
Newark, New Jersey

STEPHANIE FLICKER, M.D.

Adjunct Clinical Assistant Professor of Radiology
Thomas Jefferson University School of Medicine
Philadelphia, Pennsylvania
Chief, Department of Radiology
Deborah Heart and Lung Center
Browns Mills, New Jersey

RALPH GALLAGHER

Research Associate, Department of Surgery
Newark Beth Israel Medical Center
Newark, New Jersey

DRYDEN MORSE, M.D.

Clinical Associate Professor of Thoracic Surgery
Rutgers Medical School
Director, Pacemaker Clinic
Deborah Heart and Lung Center
Browns Mills, New Jersey

VICTOR PARSONNET, M.D.

Director of Surgery
Director of the Pacemaker Clinic and the Pacemaker Foundation
Newark Beth Israel Medical Center
Newark, New Jersey

ROBERT M. STEINER, M.D.

Professor of Radiology
Associate Professor of Medicine
Chief, Thoracic Radiology
Thomas Jefferson University School of Medicine
Philadelphia, Pennsylvania

CHARLES J. TEGTMEYER, M.D.

Professor of Radiology
Associate Professor of Anatomy
Director of Angiography and Special Procedures
University of Virginia School of Medicine
Charlottesville, Virginia

CONTENTS

1 THE RADIOLOGY OF CARDIAC PACEMAKERS—
   UPDATE   S-1

   ROBERT M. STEINER, M.D., STEPHANIE FLICKER, M.D., and CHARLES
   TEGTMEYER, M.D.

2 PACEMAKER ATLAS   S-11

   DRYDEN MORSE, M.D.

3 LEADS AND ELECTRODES   S-135

   VICTOR PARSONNET, M.D., ALAN D. BERNSTEIN, Eng.Sc.D., and RALPH
   GALLAGHER

4 LIST OF CONNECTOR SIZES FOR VARIOUS PACEMAKER
   MODELS   S-143

   VICTOR PARSONNET, M.D., ALAN D. BERNSTEIN, Eng.Sc.D., and RALPH
   GALLAGHER

5 LEAD ATLAS   S-147

   VICTOR PARSONNET, M.D., ALAN D. BERNSTEIN, Eng.Sc.D., and RALPH
   GALLAGHER

APPENDIX. ADDRESSES AND TELEPHONE NUMBERS OF
MANUFACTURERS   S-199

INDEX   S-201

.

CHAPTER 1

THE RADIOLOGY OF CARDIAC PACEMAKERS—UPDATE

Robert M. Steiner, M.D., Stephanie Flicker, M.D., and Charles Tegtmeyer, M.D.

Diagnostic imaging techniques and the diagnostic radiologist have an increasingly important task in identifying,[1–5] documenting,[6] and sometimes correcting[7,8] the complications of pacemaker and other cardiac electronic apparatus implantation.[9] Radiology also plays an ancillary role in guiding the initial implantation surgery and monitoring the outcome of the procedure. Recently, both ionizing radiation in high doses and superconducting magnetic fields used in magnetic resonance imaging have been found to damage or alter the function of modern pacemakers.[10–13]

In the following discussion, new developments in the role of radiology in cardiac pacemaker technology are considered. The possibility of a deleterious effect of ionizing radiation on pacemaker circuitry was considered in the past.[14] Studies by Hilder, Linhart, and Poole,[15] for example, demonstrated that ionizing radiation caused no alterations in pacemaker function in the therapeutic range when P-wave synchronous and ventricular-demand pacers were exposed to a total dose of 460 Gy (1 Gy = 100 rads) using cobalt-60 gamma radiation. Walz and coworkers[16] showed that there was no significant deleterious effect on five different demand pacemakers after high doses of radiation from cobalt-60, linear accelerator, and betatron therapy.

However, Marbach and associates[12] found altered function in four types of demand pacemakers after 120 Gy. It was felt that the metal oxide semiconductors now used were more sensitive to ionizing radiation than the older bipolar leads discussed in earlier papers.[14–16]

Pacemakers with metal oxide circuitry demonstrated a 10 percent decrease in pulse rate after receiving as little as 70 to 90 Gy using cobalt-60. The pacemaker with metal oxide circuitry became nonfunctional after 120 Gy.[10–11] In this series, ionizing radiation did not affect circuitry that did not contain metal oxide. It is important to consider that doses below 70 Gy did not decrease the pulse rate so that the presence of the pacemaker was not a contraindication to radiation therapy in most patients receiving cobalt therapy. Betatron- and linear accelerator–derived ionizing radiation had the effect of temporarily reducing pacemaker inhibitory function owing to the ambient electromagnetic fields of the betatron and linear accelerator, causing closing of the reed delay switch so that continuous pacing resulted. After the magnetic fields were removed, normal function was restored.[10,13]

Quertermous and colleagues[10] described an example of permanent pulse generator failure with a ''runaway'' rhythm after 21 Gy of photon radiation with a linear accelerator given to a programmable A-V sequential pacer (Intermedics Cyberlith 259-01). Damage to the metal oxide circuitry was found. A similar experience occurred with unit failure at 30 to 36 Gy, thought to be due to particle damage to the integrated circuitry of the pulse generator, leading to internodal circuit leakage causing aberrant function.[11]

It seems reasonable to monitor patients receiving therapeutic doses of ionizing radiation continuously with electrocardiography during treatment and when feasible move the generator to a location beyond the radiation portal. Needless to say, additional study is necessary to determine the precise limits of radiation therapy needed to cause pacemaker dysfunction.

THE EFFECT OF MAGNETIC RESONANCE

In addition to the electromagnetic effects of therapeutic levels of betatron and linear accelerator radiation on pacemaker function,[10-12] the effect of magnetic resonance on pacemaker activity is a limiting factor in the use of this new imaging modality in diagnosis.[13] Whereas large static magnetic fields (up to 2 T*) used to orient hydrogen atoms have not been associated with harmful effects on human tissue, time-varying gradient fields and radiofrequency pulses used to re-orient proton spins may present problems for implanted metallic devices.[17] The initiator of the activity of the reed switch, closed to bypass the pacemaker sensing system and convert the pacemaker to asynchronous operation for patient analysis, is an external hand-held magnet of approximately 0.1 T. Thus, pacemakers placed in the magnetic field of a magnetic resonance imaging unit revert to an asynchronous mode because the reed switch closes. As a result, the pacer is unresponsive to electromagnetic interference or signals from time-varying magnetic fields that simulate cardiac activity.[13]

If the demand pacer does not have a functioning reed switch, electromagnetic interference can simulate normal electric activity unless protective measures such as stainless-steel shielding and pulse frequency and amplitude discrimination are built into the pacemaker system. Time-varying magnetic resonance fields may induce a voltage signal in the pacer lead that may mimic the pulse width and repetition rate of the normal cardiac cycle and can be recognized as cardiac activity by the pacer's circuitry.

Various ferromagnetic components of the pacemaker may be affected by time-varying magnetic fields. The force of attraction and torque are dependent on the distance between the pacemaker generator and the magnetic resonance imager. Torque will occur when the generator aligns itself along the magnetic field lines. Theoretically, the pacemaker may turn within the surgical pocket if adequate space permits.[13]

In a study by Pavlicek and coworkers[13] of six demand pacemakers of different manufacturers, closure of the reed switch occurred with a minimum of 17 gauss at a distance of 5.4 m from a 0.5-T superconducting magnetic resonance instrument—a commonly used field strength. The sensitivity varied depending on the orientation of the pacemaker, up to a maximum of 730 gauss. Two of the six pacemakers showed sufficient torque to result in significant motion within the pacemaker pocket.[13] It is thought that after analysis of the magnetic resonance effect on the six pacemakers, an acceptable limit for access to a magnetic resonance imager is 10 gauss.[13]

PACEMAKER IMPLANTATION

Although the radiographic appearance of normal pacemaker implantation is well described,[18,19] the position of the right atrial (RA) lead used alone or in conjunction with

---

* T = tesla

right ventricular (RV) pacing needs emphasis.[4] The right atrial appendage (RAA) is a deep muscular pocket in the superior anterior aspect of the right atrium. Its shape and position allow for stable and rapid implantation.

A correctly placed RAA lead projects anteriorly and upward on the lateral chest radiograph, and cephalad and slightly to the right or left on the frontal projection. On fluoroscopy, the lead sways back and forth and left to right with each contraction of the atrium.[5] Increasing use of RAA leads is due to recognition of the hemodynamic dependence of the contribution of atrial systole to cardiac output in patients with active lives who require the increased heart rate capability of atrial-demand pacing during exercise and in patients in whom a sudden loss of atrioventricular synchrony leads to hypotension and syncope.[4]

The value of two-dimensional echocardiography in monitoring pacemaker insertion as well as its value in identifying malposition, displacement, and perforation is well described.[21] The importance of this technique should be emphasized with patients in intensive care units, children, women in the childbearing age-group, and others for whom fluoroscopy and/or posteroanterior and lateral plain films of the chest are difficult to obtain or detrimental. Particularly in perforation of the right ventricle, with or without hemopericardium, two-dimensional echocardiography is superior to plain film technique and diagnosis. A disadvantage of echocardiography is the need for careful examination in multiple planes since the entire catheter is not seen in a single plane. In addition, the pacing lead may be confused with other intracardiac catheters or with intracardiac structures such as trabeculae or chordae.[3]

Rapid-acquisition cardiovascular computed tomography (RACVCT) (Imatron C-100) is also a useful technique in identifying the location of implanted pacemaker leads. A short exposure time of 50 msec, together with ECG gating and a programmed cine display mode, allows for excellent depiction of cardiac anatomy following contrast enhancement.

Areas of asynergy or aneurysm in the area of pacemaker lead fixation and the normal position of the lead thought to be malpositioned in a patient with marked cardiomegaly are examples of the value of this technique (Fig. 1-1). Although RACVCT is less invasive than angiography, it has the disadvantage of relatively high radiation dose, unlike echocardiography.[2]

EXTRACTION OF INTRAVASCULAR PACEMAKER LEADS

As more transvenous tined and corkscrew leads, developed to ensure adequate fixation to the endocardium, are left in place after the generator is removed, problems have arisen that are the subject of an expanding medical literature. These leads may migrate on occasion from their positions in the subclavian vein to other intravascular positions. This may occur if the proximal end of the lead is not adequately secured when the generator is removed and when the electrode in the right ventricle becomes dislodged.[5,7,8]

Although leads may be extracted transvenously with angiographic catheters or snares (Fig. 1-2), occasionally open surgery is needed to remove the catheter. Removal is particularly important if infective endocarditis is diagnosed.[7,8,22] Although successful treatment of pacemaker infection has occurred when the old generator is removed, as in a case reported by Schwartz and associates,[7] an active vegetation remained on the extracted catheter removed in a patient apparently well after antibiotic treatment. This example suggests that the catheter as well as the generator should be removed if possible in patients treated for pacemaker-related infective endocarditis.[7]

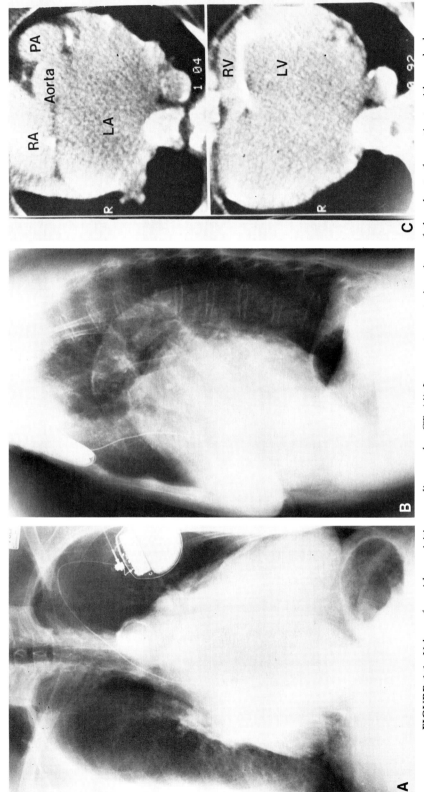

FIGURE 1-1. Value of rapid-acquisition cardiovascular CT. (*A*) In a posteroanterior view of the chest of a patient with marked cardiomegaly, the pacemaker lead appears to lie in an abnormal position above and to the left of the right ventricular apex. (*B*) In the lateral view of the chest, the distal tip of the lead lies above the area of the right ventricular apex. (*C*) Rapid-acquisition cardiovascular CT following contrast enhancement clearly defines the unusual pathway of the catheter. The enlarged left ventricle displaces the right ventricle forward and cephalad. The catheter lies in normal position in the right ventricle apex (RA = right atrium; PA = pulmonary artery; LV = left ventricular artery; RV = right ventricle; arrow = catheter).

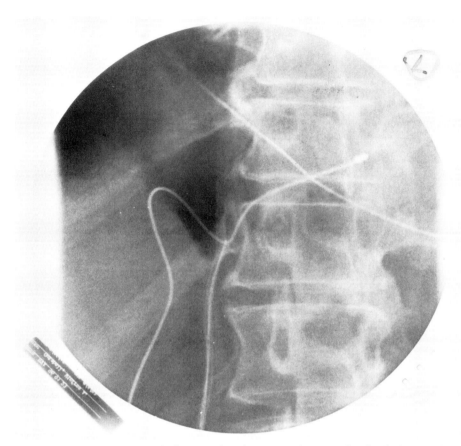

FIGURE 1-2. Transvenous retrieval of retained malpositioned pacemaker lead. A snare introduced following a right ventricular venous puncture is secured around the pacemaker lead. The lead was withdrawn into the iliac vein and removed following a venous cutdown.

AUTOMATIC IMPLANTABLE CARDIOVERTER-DEFIBRILLATOR

In the United States, sudden death from ventricular tachyarrhythmias (VTA) occurs in almost 0.5 million people each year. Patients who experience VTA have a high recurrence rate, and the expected mortality 1 year from recurrence is 35 to 45 percent.[9]

To alleviate this sword of Damocles, the automatic implantable cardioverter-defibrillator (AICD, Intec Systems) detects VTA and responds by delivering a cardioverting or defibrillating shock to the heart from an implanted system.[23] The AICD, which superficially resembles a transvenous pacemaker, is of interest to the imaging diagnostician because initial insertion and potential complications associated with this apparatus should be similar to those associated with cardiac pacemakers, including component fracture, lead dislodgment, and infection.

The AICD consists of electronics and lithium-iodide batteries encased in titanium. A microprocessor monitors cardiac rhythm and detects ventricular tachycardia (VT) or ventricular fibrillation (VF). The rate-monitoring electrode consists of either a pair of epicardial electrodes screwed into the left ventricular myocardium or right ventricular endocardial bipolar electrodes.[9] The shocking leads are either a spring-patch or a patch-patch electrode configuration. The anode is in the superior vena cava or right atrium and is used in conjunction with the epicardial patch electrode placed in the left ventricular apex or the left ventricular lateral wall.

When the patch-patch system is used, the spring anode is replaced by a patch applied to the anterior right ventricle facing the ventricle patch. The electronic canister is placed in a subcutaneous pouch in the anterior abdominal wall.

The most common complication seen radiographically appears to be migration of the spring lead,[1,9] seen in three of 25 patients in Goodman and associates' series.[9] No similar problems were observed with the patch-patch configuration.

REFERENCES

1. VELTRI, EP, MOWER, MM, and REID, PR: *Twiddler's syndrome: A new twist.* PACE 7:1004–1009, 1984.
2. FLICKER, S, ELDREDGE, WJ, NAIDECH, HJ, STEINER, RM, and CLARK, DL: *Computed tomographic localization of malposition of pacing electrodes: The value of cardiovascular computed tomography.* PACE 8:589–599, July-August 1985.
3. TOBIN, AM, GRODMAN, RS, FISHER, A, KELLER, M, and NICOLOSI, R: *Two-dimensional echocardiographic localization of a malpositioned pacing catheter.* PACE 6:291–299, 1983.
4. HERTZBERG, BS, CHILES, C, and RAVIN, CE: *Right atrial appendage pacing: Radiographic considerations.* AJR 145:31–34, 1985.
5. WIDMANN, WD, EDOGA, JK, GARFRAS, D, and MCLEAN, ER: *Peripheral migration of pacemaker electrodes.* PACE 7:227–229, 1984.
6. FELICE, R, HUTTON, L, and KLEIN, G: *Cardiac pacemaker leads—a radiographic perspective.* J Can Assoc Radiol 35:20–23, 1984.
7. SCHWARTZ, AB, FUNG, G, LEWIS, A, HUNTER, G, VERLENDEN, W, and KLANSNER, S: *Extraction of an intravascularized pacemaker lead—a new approach to an unusual problem.* PACE 7:999–1003, 1984.
8. MARSCH, B, ERTL, G, and KULKE, H: *Extraction of a chronically infected endocardial screw-in pacemaker lead by pigtail catheter and wire loop via the femoral vein.* PACE 8:230–234, 1985.
9. GOODMAN, LR, TROUP, PJ, THORSEN, MK, and YOUKER, JE: *Automatic implantable cardioverter-defibrillator: Radiographic appearance.* Radiology 155:571–573, 1985.
10. QUERTERMOUS, T, MEGAHY, MS, DAS GUPTA, DS, and GRIEN, ML: *Pacemaker failure resulting from radiation damage.* Radiology 148:257–258, 1983.
11. KATZENBERG, CA, MARCUS, FL, HEUSINKVELD, RS, and MAMMANA, RB: *Pacemaker failure due to radiation therapy.* PACE 5:156–159, 1982.
12. MARBACH, JR, MEOZ-MENDEZ, RT, HUFFMAN, JK, HUDGINS, PT, and ALMOND, PR: *The effects on cardiac pacemakers of ionizing radiation and electromagnetic interference from radiotherapy machines.* Int J Radiat Oncol Biol Phys 4:1055–1058, 1978.
13. PAVLICEK, W, GEISINGER, M, CASTLE, L, BORKOWSKI, GP, MEANY, TF, BREAM, BL, and GALLAGHER, JH: *The effects of Nuclear Magnetic Resonance on patients with cardiac pacemakers.* Radiology 147:149–153, 1983.
14. SMYTH, NPD, PARSONNET, V, ESCHER, DJW, and FURMAN, S: *The pacemaker patient and the electromagnetic environment.* JAMA 227:1412, 1974.
15. HILDER, FJ, LINHART, JW, and POOLE, DO: *Irradiation of pulmonary tumor with overlying artificial cardiac pacemaker.* Radiology 92:148–149, 1969.
16. WALZ, BJ, REDER, RE, PASTORE, JO, LITTMAN, P, and JOHNSON, R: *Cardiac pacemakers: Does radiation therapy affect performance?* JAMA 234:72–73, 1975.
17. BUDINGER, TF: *Nuclear Magnetic Resonance (NMR) in vivo studies: Known thresholds for health effects.* J Comput Assist Tomogr 5:800–811, 1981.
18. STEINER, RM and MORSE, D: *The radiology of cardiac pacemakers.* JAMA 240:2574–2578, 1978.
19. HEWITT, MJ, CHEN, JTT, RAVIN, CT, and GALLAGHER, JJ: *Coronary sinus atrial pacing: Radiographic considerations.* AJR 136:323–328, 1981.
20. BYRD, C: *Permanent pacemaker implantation techniques.* In Samet, P and El-Sherif, N (eds): *Cardiac Pacing,* ed 2. Grune & Stratton, New York, 1980, pp 229–253.

21. NANDA, NC: *Evaluation of pacing function by real time two-dimensional echocardiography.* Impulse 17:2–5, 1980.
22. CHOO, MH, HOLMES, DR, and GERSH, BJ: *Permanent pacemaker infections: Characterization and management.* Am J Cardiol 48:559, 1981.
23. MIROWSKI, M, REID, PR, and MOWER, MM: *Termination of malignant ventricular arrhythmias with an implanted automatic defibrillator in human beings.* N Engl J Med 303:322–324, 1980.

CHAPTER 2

PACEMAKER ATLAS

Dryden Morse, M.D.

TABLE OF CONTENTS—PACEMAKERS AND ANCILLARY EQUIPMENT

COMPANY	MODEL	PAGE
Biotronik	Diplos 04	S-12
	Diplos 05	S-14
	Kalos 03-1	S-16
	Kalos 04	S-18
	Neos 01-1	S-20
	Neos M 01-1	S-22
	Leptos 01-1	S-24
	EDP-20 External Generator	S-26
	EPR-500 Programmer	S-28
	EDP-30 Dual-Chamber External Generator	S-30
Cardiac Control Systems, Inc.	105 Maestro	S-32
	501 Maestro	S-34
	1000 Maestro Programmer	S-36
Cardiac Pacemakers, Inc.	Astra 6 429/529	S-38
	Ultra I 531/631/635	S-40
	Ultra II 910	S-42
	Delta 925	S-44
	2030 Programmer	S-46
	2035 Hand-Held Programmer/Printer	S-48
	2040 Programmer	S-50
Cardio-Pace Medical	Durapulse P101 Unipolar, P102 Bipolar	S-52
	1000 Programmer	S-55
Cordis	Sequicor II, Model 233F	S-56
	Sequicor III, Models 233G/ GR/GL	S-58

COMPANY	MODEL	PAGE
	Multicor γ (Gamma), Models 336A/B and 337A	S-60
	Multicor II, Models 402A/B/C	S-62
	Gemini θ (Theta), Model 415A	S-64
	Gemini III, Model 418A	S-66
	297A Chronocor V External Pacer External Generator	S-68
	Cordis Computer-Driven, Dual-Channel Electrophysiology (EP) Stimulator	S-70
ELA Medical	Multilith 2 1250 Monopolar/ 2250 Bipolar	S-72
	Unilith 2 (7550)	S-74
Intermedics	Prima 235-01	S-76
	SuPrima 253-21	S-78
	Quantum 254-20	S-80
	Galaxy 271-03	S-82
	Nova 281-01	S-84
	Cosmos 283-01 (unipolar)/ Cosmos 284-02 (bipolar)	S-86
	320-02 ''Pocket Programmer''	S-88
	522-06 Programmer	S-90
Medtronic, Inc.	Byrel-SX, Model 5993-SX	S-92
	Versatrax II, Model 7000A	S-94
	Symbios 7005 dual unipolar, 7005C dual universal unipolar, 7006 dual bipolar	S-96
	Symbios, Model 7008	S-98
	Pasys, Models 8320, 8322, 8326, 8328, and 8329	S-100
	Activitrax, Models 8400, 8402, and 8403	S-102
	Classix, Models 8436E, 8437E, 8438C	S-104
	5311-A-V Pacing System Analyzer	S-106
	5320 External Generator	S-108
	5326 Programmable Stimulator for Cardiac Electrophysiologic Studies	S-110
	5330 Dual-Chamber External Generator	S-112
	5375 Demand Pulse Generator	S-114
	9710 Programmer and Printer	S-116
Pacesetter Systems, Inc.	223 Programalith AV	S-118
	225/226 Programalith II	S-120
	241/242 Programalith III	S-122
	261/262	S-124
	AFP Series 273/275/281/283	S-126

COMPANY	MODEL	PAGE
Siemens-Elema	688	S-128
	Dialog AV 704	S-130
Vitatron Medical B.V.	Ceryx 6, Model 611/Ceryx 3, Model 311	S-132

BIOTRONIK

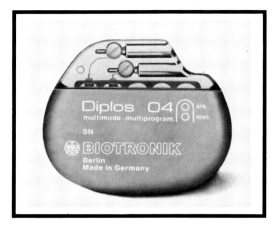 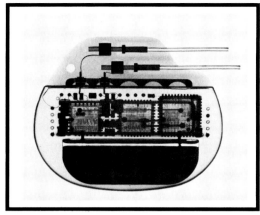

1. IDENTIFICATION/INFORMATION

Model:	Diplos 04
24-Hr Telephone Number:	1-800-547-0394
Method of Operation (ICHD code):	DDD
Cost:	$4775 (tentative)

2. SPECIAL FEATURES

3. PROGRAMMABLE FEATURES

Rate:	31, 41, 51, 62, 72, 82, 92 ppm
DOO, VOO, AOO:	113 ppm
Amplitude:	A & V = 2.5, 5.0 V
Pulse Duration (width):	A & V = 0.13, 0.25, 0.5, 1.0 msec
Sensitivity:	A (15 msec) = 0.6, 1.2, 2.0; V (40 msec) = 1.6, 2.4, 4.8 msec
Refractory:	A = 300, 350, 400, 450, 500; V = 300, 400 msec
Hysteresis:	off, 10 ppm, AT 62, 72, 82, 92 ppm
AV Delay:	15, 50, 100, 125, 150, 175, 200, 250, 300 msec
Changes of Mode (e.g., VVT to VVI):	DDD, DVI, VDD, COM/UNCOM, DAT, DOO, VAT, VVI, VOO, AAI, AOO
Telemetry Response:	bidirectional—500 programmer
AV Fallback:	0, 40, 50, 60 msec
Tachycardia Response:	2:1 block: or Wenckebach
Upper Tracking Rate:	100, 125, 150, 171 ppm
Runaway Protection:	A = 130 ppm, V = upper tracking rate

4. ELECTRICAL CHARACTERISTICS

5. POWER SOURCE

Number of Cells:	1
Manufacturer/Model Number:	CRC 908
Major Chemicals:	LiI_2
Capacity:	1.9 amp-hr

6. LONGEVITY INFORMATION

Warranty:	50 mo

7. POWER SOURCE DEPLETION INDICATOR

Change in Pulse Rate:	11% decrease

8. METHOD FOR PERIODIC TEST OF PROPER FUNCTION

Magnet Test Rate:	programmed rate
Orientation of Magnet or Programmer:	apply and remove vertically to pacer
Does Magnet Work if Pacer Is Upside Down:	yes
Is Special Magnet Required:	no

9. **EFFECT OF ELECTRICAL AND MAGNETIC FIELDS**

10. **PHYSICAL CHARACTERISTICS**

Dimensions (mm):	$62 \times 53 \times 11.5$
Weight (g):	56
Material in Contact With Tissue:	titanium

11. **NONINVASIVE IDENTIFICATION:** no radiopaque letters

12. **TERMINAL CONNECTOR COMPATIBILITY**

Cordis Lead:	no
Medtronic Lead:	yes
Unipolar:	yes
Accepts Atrial and Ventricular:	yes

13. **TELEMETRY**

All Programmed Parameters:	yes

BIOTRONIK

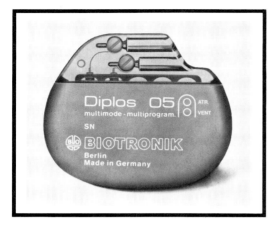 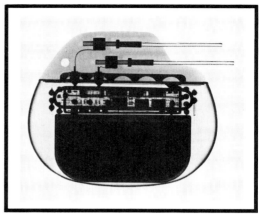

1. IDENTIFICATION/INFORMATION

Model:	Diplos 05
24-Hr Telephone Number:	1-800-547-0394
Method of Operation (ICHD code):	DDD
Cost:	$4975 (tentative)

2. SPECIAL FEATURES

3. PROGRAMMABLE FEATURES

Rate:	32, 41, 51, 62, 72, 82, 92 ppm (DOO, VOO, AOO: 113 ppm)
Amplitude:	A & V = 2.5, 5.0 V
Pulse Duration (width):	A & V = 0.13, 0.25, 0.5, 1.0 msec
Sensitivity:	A 0.6, 1.2, 2.0 mV; V 1.6, 2.4, 4.8 mV
Refractory:	A = 300, 350, 400, 450, 500; V = 300, 400 msec
Hysteresis:	off, 10 ppm at 62, 72, 82, 92 ppm
AV Delay:	15, 50, 100, 125, 150, 175, 200, 250, 300 msec
Changes of Mode (e.g., VVT to VVI):	DOO, DVI, VDD, COM/UNCOM, DAT, DOO, VAT, VVI, VOO, AAI, AOO
Telemetry Response:	bidirectional—500 programmer
Other:	AV fallback—0, 40, 50, 60 msec

4. ELECTRICAL CHARACTERISTICS

Sensitivity (mV):	tachycardia response: 2:1 block or Wenckebach
Pulse Duration (width):	upper tracking rate: 100, 125, 150, 171 ppm
Pulse Amplitude (V):	(see above)
Upper Rate Limits:	A = 130 ppm; V = upper tracking rate

5. POWER SOURCE

Number of Cells:	1
Manufacturer/Model Number:	CRC 920
Major Chemicals:	lithium iodine
Capacity:	2.8 amp-hr

6. LONGEVITY INFORMATION

Warranty:	lifetime
Manufacturer's Projected Life:	95 mo

7. POWER SOURCE DEPLETION INDICATOR

Change in Pulse Rate:	11% decrease

8. METHOD FOR PERIODIC TEST OF PROPER FUNCTION

Magnet Test Rate:	programmed rate
Orientation of Magnet or Programmer:	apply and remove vertically to pacer

Does Magnet Work if Pacer Is Upside Down: yes
Is Special Magnet Required: no

9. EFFECT OF ELECTRICAL AND MAGNETIC FIELDS

10. PHYSICAL CHARACTERISTICS

Dimensions (mm): $62 \times 53 \times 11.5$
Weight (g):   58
Material in Contact With Tissue: titanium

11. NONINVASIVE IDENTIFICATION

Other: see x-ray

12. TERMINAL CONNECTOR COMPATIBILITY

Cordis Lead: no
Medtronic Lead: yes
Unipolar: yes
Accepts Atrial and Ventricular: yes

BIOTRONIK

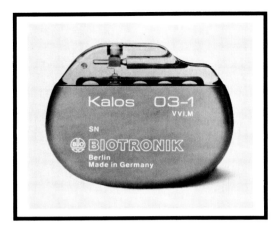 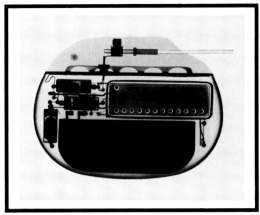

1. IDENTIFICATION/INFORMATION

Model:	Kalos 03-1
24-Hr Telephone Number:	1-800-547-0394; 1-503-635-3594
Method of Operation (ICHD code):	VVI, M

2. SPECIAL FEATURES

3. PROGRAMMABLE FEATURES

Rate:	31, 41, 51, 62, 72, 82, 92, 113 = VOO
Amplitude:	4.8 V, 7.3 V
Pulse Duration (width):	0.13, 0.25, 0.5, 1.0
Sensitivity:	1.4, 3.2 mV
Hysteresis:	off, 10 ppm at 62, 72, 82, 92 ppm
Changes of Mode (e.g., VVT to VVI):	VVI, VOO

4. ELECTRICAL CHARACTERISTICS

Basic Rate (ppm):	72
Refractory Period:	300 msec
Upper Rate Limit; Run Away:	130 ppm

5. POWER SOURCE

Number of Cells:	1
Manufacturer/Model Number:	CRC 906 or WG 8031
Major Chemicals:	lithium iodine
Capacity:	normal 1.7 amp-hr or 1.9 amp-hr

6. LONGEVITY INFORMATION

Warranty:	95 mo
Manufacturer's Projected Life:	95 mo or 101 mo

7. POWER SOURCE DEPLETION INDICATOR

Change in Pulse Rate:	6% programmed rate

8. METHOD FOR PERIODIC TEST OF PROPER FUNCTION

9. EFFECT OF ELECTRICAL AND MAGNETIC FIELDS

10. PHYSICAL CHARACTERISTICS

Dimensions (mm):	62 × 48 × 8.8
Weight (g):	49
Material in Contact With Tissue:	titanium

11. NONINVASIVE IDENTIFICATION

Other:	none

12. TERMINAL CONNECTOR COMPATIBILITY

Cordis Lead:	Model 104-1B unipolar
Medtronic Lead:	Model 104-1A unipolar
Bipolar:	Model 129-ABP

13. TELEMETRY

BIOTRONIK

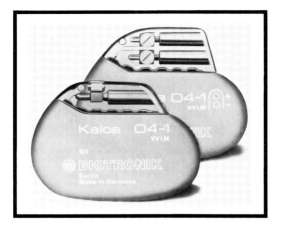 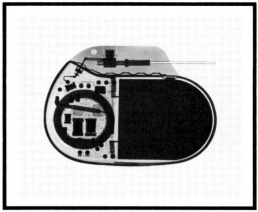

1. IDENTIFICATION/INFORMATION

Model:	Kalos 04
24-Hr Telephone Number:	1-800-547-0394
Method of Operation (ICHD code):	VVI, VOO
Cost:	$3575

2. SPECIAL FEATURES

3. PROGRAMMABLE FEATURES

Rate:	31, 41, 51, 62, 72, 82, 92 ppm; VOO = 113 ppm
Amplitude:	4.8, 7.3 V
Pulse Duration (width):	0.13, 0.25, 0.5, 1.0 msec
Sensitivity:	1.4, 3.2 mV
Other:	use model 400 or 500 programmer

4. ELECTRICAL CHARACTERISTICS

Magnet Rate (ppm):	= programmed rate
Refractory Period:	300 msec
Upper Rate Limit; Run Away:	130 ppm

5. POWER SOURCE

Number of Cells:	1
Manufacturer/Model Number:	CRC 912 or WG 8206
Major Chemicals:	LiI_2
Capacity:	2.0 amp-hr

6. LONGEVITY INFORMATION

Warranty:	109 mo
Manufacturer's Projected Life:	109 mo

7. POWER SOURCE DEPLETION INDICATOR

Change in Pulse Rate:	6% decrease

8. METHOD FOR PERIODIC TEST OF PROPER FUNCTION

Magnet Test Rate:	programmed rate
Orientation of Magnet or Programmer:	apply and remove vertically to pacer
Does Magnet Work if Pacer Is Upside Down:	yes
Is Special Magnet Required:	no

9. EFFECT OF ELECTRICAL AND MAGNETIC FIELDS

10. PHYSICAL CHARACTERISTICS

Dimensions (mm):	57 × 41 × 8.8
Weight (g):	37
Material:	titanium

11. NONINVASIVE IDENTIFICATION: no code

12. TERMINAL CONNECTOR COMPATIBILITY

Cordis Lead:	Model 907-1B unipolar
Medtronic Lead:	Model 900-1A unipolar
Bipolar:	Model 922-ABP

BIOTRONIK

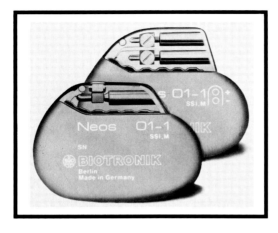 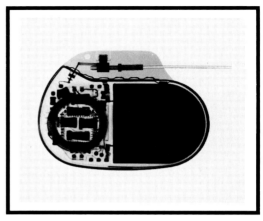

1. IDENTIFICATION/INFORMATION

Model:	Neos 01-1
24-Hr Telephone Number:	1-800-547-0394
Method of Operation (ICHD code):	VVI, AAI, VOO, AOO
Cost:	$4375

2. SPECIAL FEATURES

3. PROGRAMMABLE FEATURES

Rate:	30, 40, 50, 55, 60, 70, 75, 80, 85, 90, 100, 110
Amplitude:	2.4, 3.1, 3.6, 4.8, 6.2, 7.2, 9.6 V
Pulse Duration (width):	0.25, 0.5, 0.75, 1.0 msec
Sensitivity:	0.8, 1.6, 2.4, 3.2, 4.0, 4.8, 5.6 mV
Refractory:	250, 300, 350, 400 msec
Hysteresis:	off, 40, 50, 60 ppm
Changes of Mode (e.g., VVT to VVI):	VVI, VOO, AAI, AOO
Telemetry Response:	bidirectional
Other:	noninvasive stimulation threshold, 400 or 500 programmer

4. ELECTRICAL CHARACTERISTICS

Upper Rate Limit; Run Away:	130 ppm

5. POWER SOURCE

Number of Cells:	1
Manufacturer/Model Number:	CRC 912 or WG 8206
Major Chemicals:	lithium iodine
Capacity:	2.0 amp-hr

6. LONGEVITY INFORMATION

Warranty:	lifetime
Manufacturer's Projected Life:	104 mo

7. POWER SOURCE DEPLETION INDICATOR

Change in Pulse Rate:	11% decrease
Change in Pulse Amplitude:	stays constant

8. METHOD FOR PERIODIC TEST OF PROPER FUNCTION

Magnet Test Rate:	same as programmed
Orientation of Magnet and Programmer:	apply and remove vertically to pacer
Does Magnet Work if Pacer Is Upside Down:	yes
Is Special Magnet Required:	no

9. EFFECT OF ELECTRICAL AND MAGNETIC FIELDS

10. PHYSICAL CHARACTERISTICS

Dimensions (mm):	57 × 41 × 8.8

Weight (g): 37
Material in Contact With Tissue: titanium

11. NONINVASIVE IDENTIFICATION
X-ray Code (radiopaque letters): none

12. TERMINAL CONNECTOR COMPATIBILITY
Cordis Lead: Model 125-2B unipolar
Medtronic Lead: Model 125-2A unipolar
Bipolar: Model 160 ABP

13. TELEMETRY: bidirectional

BIOTRONIK

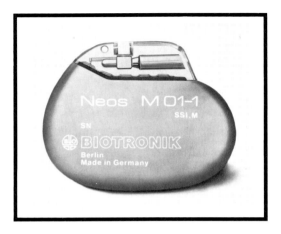 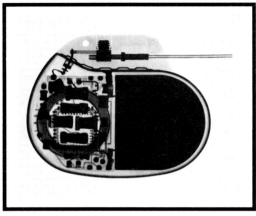

1. IDENTIFICATION/INFORMATION

Model:	Neos M 01-1
24-Hr Telephone Number:	1-800-547-0394
Method of Operation (ICHD code):	VVI, AAI, VOO, AOO
Cost:	$3775

2. SPECIAL FEATURES: Small, light, multiprogrammable with telemetry

3. PROGRAMMABLE FEATURES

Rate:	30, 40, 50, 55, 60, 70, 80, 85, 90, 100, 110
Amplitude:	2.4, 3.1, 3.6, 4.8, 6.2, 7.2, 9.6 V
Pulse Duration (width):	0.25, 0.5, 0.75, 1.0 msec
Sensitivity:	0.8, 1.6, 2.4, 3.2, 4.0, 4.8, 5.6 mV
Refractory:	250, 300, 350, 400 msec
Hysteresis:	off, 40, 50, 60 ppm
AV Delay:	N/A
Changes of Mode (e.g., VVT to VVI):	VVI, AAI, VOO, AOO
Telemetry Response:	bidirectional
Other:	noninvasive stimulation threshold test. Note: Use model 400 or 500 programmers

4. ELECTRICAL CHARACTERISTICS

Upper Rate Limit; Run Away:	130 ppm

5. POWER SOURCE

Number of Cells:	1
Manufacturer/Model Number:	CRC 914 or WG 8207
Major Chemicals:	LiI_2
Capacity:	1.6 amp-hr

6. LONGEVITY INFORMATION

Warranty:	82 mo
Manufacturer's Projected Life:	82 mo

7. POWER SOURCE DEPLETION INDICATOR

Change in Pulse Rate:	11% decrease
Pulse Width:	stays constant
Pulse Amplitude:	stays constant

8. METHOD FOR PERIODIC TEST OF PROPER FUNCTION

Magnet Test Rate:	same as programmed
Orientation of Magnet or Programmer:	apply and remove vertically to pacer
Does Magnet Work if Pacer Is Upside Down:	yes
Is Special Magnet Required:	no

9. EFFECT OF ELECTRICAL AND MAGNETIC FIELDS

10. PHYSICAL CHARACTERISTICS

Dimensions (mm):	$51 \times 41 \times 8.8$
Weight (g):	31
Material in Contact With Tissue:	titanium

11. NONINVASIVE IDENTIFICATION

X-ray Code (radiopaque letters):   no radiopaque letters; shorter battery length

12. TERMINAL CONNECTOR COMPATIBILITY

Cordis Lead:	164-2B unipolar
Medtronic Lead:	164-2A unipolar
Unipolar:	yes

13. TELEMETRY: bidirectional telemetric system documents interrogated program and measured rate and pulse width.

BIOTRONIK

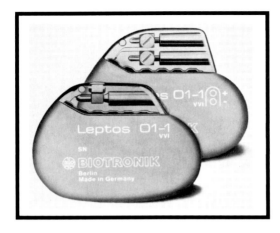
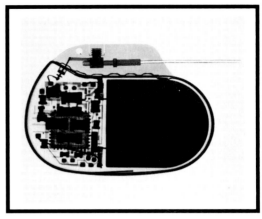

1. IDENTIFICATION/INFORMATION

Model:	Leptos 01-1
24-Hr Telephone Number:	1-800-547-0394
Method of Operation (ICHD code):	VVI
Cost:	$1675

2. SPECIAL FEATURES

3. PROGRAMMABLE FEATURES: not programmable

4. ELECTRICAL CHARACTERISTICS

Sensitivity (mV):	2.4
Pulse Duration (width):	0.5 msec
Pulse Amplitude (V):	4.8
Basic Rate (ppm):	70
Magnet Rate (ppm):	70
Refractory Period:	300 msec
Upper Rate Limit:	run away 130 ppm

5. POWER SOURCE

Number of Cells:	1
Manufacturer/Model Number:	CRC 912 or WG 8206
Major Chemicals:	LiI_2
Capacity:	2.0 amp-hr

6. LONGEVITY INFORMATION

Warranty:	104 mo
Manufacturer's Projected Life:	104 mo

7. POWER SOURCE DEPLETION INDICATOR

Change in Pulse Rate:	11% decrease

8. METHOD FOR PERIODIC TEST OF PROPER FUNCTION

Magnet Test Rate:	70 ppm
Orientation of Magnet or Programmer:	apply and remove vertically to pacer
Does Magnet Work if Pacer Is Upside Down:	yes
Is Special Magnet Required:	no

9. EFFECT OF ELECTRICAL AND MAGNETIC FIELDS

10. PHYSICAL CHARACTERISTICS

Dimensions (mm):	57 × 41 × 8.8
Weight (g):	37
Material in Contact With Tissue:	titanium

11. NONINVASIVE IDENTIFICATION

X-ray Code (radiopaque letters):	none

12. TERMINAL CONNECTOR COMPATIBILITY*

6 mm Cordis Lead:	Model 128-1B—unipolar
5 mm Medtronic Lead:	Model 128-1B—unipolar
5 mm Bipolar:	Model 128—AOP

13. TELEMETRY: no

---

* Note: With most Biotronik pacers, three models are available. The two unipolar models have either a 5-mm or 6-mm aperture, and the bipolar unit has a 5-mm aperture.

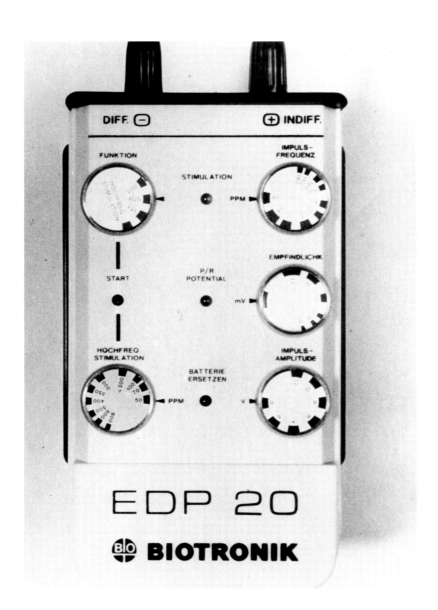

MANUFACTURER: Biotronik
MODEL: EDP-20 (Single-Chamber) External Generator

1. **Rate Range:**   40–180 ppm continuously adjustable

2. **Rate Calibration Accuracy:**   ± 5%

3. **Output Current Range:**   0–12 mA continuously adjustable

4. **Current Calibration Accuracy:**   ± 5%

5. **Pulse Width:**   0.9 msec

6. **Sensitivity Ranges:**   1–20 mV continuously adjustable (40 msec $\sin^2$ signal)

7. **Sensitivity Accuracy:**   ± 10%

8. **Refractory Period:**   250 msec

9. **Noise Rate (with EMI):**   pacing rate

10. **Power Source:**   alkaline, 9 V (e.g., Mallory Duracell MN 1604)

11. **Battery Life:**   approximately 1000 hours

12. **Physical Dimensions:**   130 × 70 × 27 mm

13. **Weight (including battery):**   250 g

14. **Material in Case:**   plastic

15. **Material in Cover:**   transparent plastic

16. **Special Features:**   Demand (VVI/AAI) and asynchronous (VOO/ADO) rapid pacing stimulation can be continuously set from 50 to as high as 800 ppm to overdrive tachycardiac rhythms; battery replacement indicator light; transparent safety cover to prevent unintentional control changes; ability to deliver up to a 12-V pulse amplitude in emergency situations. Unipolar or bipolar pacing, storage of power (10 sec) to facilitate battery changes, ability to be worn as an ambulatory device (strap included).

17. **Price:** $1575

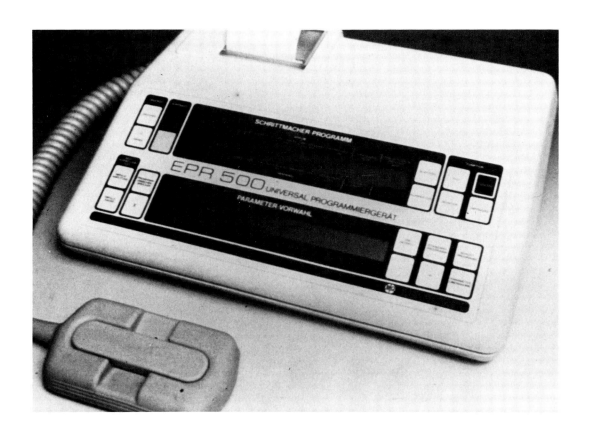

MANUFACTURER: Biotronik
MODEL: EPR-500 Programmer

1. **Carrier Frequency:**   16 kHz or 32 kHz

2. **Data Bit Transmission Rate:**   25 msec/bit or 1 msec/bit

3. **Programming Time (pulse period):**   < 2 sec

4. **Programming Range:**   within 4 cm of pacemaker face

5. **Display:**   40-position LCD display, 20-position thermal printer

6. **Programmable Parameters:**
   Rate: yes, for all programmable pacer models, by steps specific to each model
   Hysteresis: yes, for specified pacer models
   Output: yes, in volts, for specified pacer models, by steps specific to each model
   Pulse Width: yes, for specified pacer models, four steps depending on model
   Sensitivity: yes, for specified pacer models, by steps specific to each model
   Model: yes, for specified pacer model
   Refractory Period: yes, for specified pacer models, by steps specific to each model
   Telemetry: yes, for specified pacer models
   Confirm Signal: "confirmation," then "program confirmed"
   Hard Copy Printer: yes

7. **Power Source:**   110 V, 50 to 60 Hz

8. **Power Consumption:**   22 watts

9. **Operating Time:**   indefinite

10. **Pacemaker Series:**   Diplos-03, Diplos-04/05,* Nomos, Kalos, Neos-LP, Neos-M, Neos, Eikos

11. **Dimensions:**   80 × 320 × 257 mm H × W × D

12. **Weight:**   2.8 kg (16.1 lb)

13. **Special Features:**   program memory, safe (high-energy) program, standard (factory-set) program, a cursor for modifying single or multiple parameters, ability to program all programmable Biotronik pacemakers, automatic threshold test (Neos and Neos M), autoclavable plastic sheath for programming wand.

14. **Price:** $3475

---

* Currently under investigation.

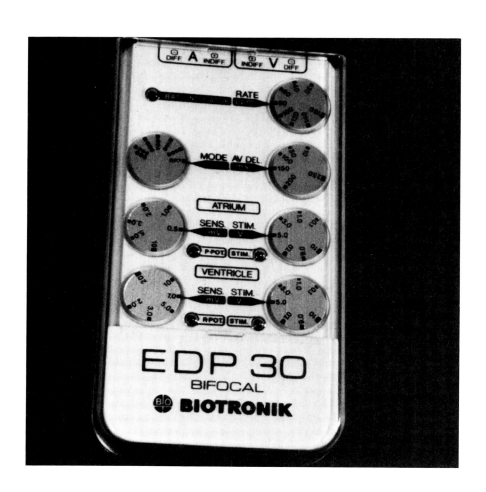

MANUFACTURER: Biotronik
MODEL: EDP-30 (Dual-Chamber) External Generator

1. **Rate Range:**   30 to 150 ppm continuously variable

2. **Rate Calibration Accuracy:**   ± 5%

3. **Output Current Range:**   variable output voltage is selectable: atrium and ventricle 0.1 to 10 V, both continuously adjustable

4. **Current Calibration Accuracy:**   N/A; voltage ± 10%

5. **Pulse Width:**   atrium 0.75 msec; ventricle 0.5 msec

6. **Sensitivity Range:**   atrium 0.5 to 10 mV (15 msec-sin²-signal); ventricle 2 to 20 mV (40 msec-sin²-signal); both continuously adjustable

7. **Sensitivity Accuracy:**   ± 10%

8. **Refractory Period:**   atrium: 400 to 500 msec; ventricle: 225 msec

9. **Noise Rate (with EMI):**   pacing rate

10. **Power Source:**   alkaline cell 9 V (e.g., Mallory MN 1604)

11. **Battery Life:**   approximately 400 hours

12. **Physical Dimensions:**   130 × 70 × 23 mm

13. **Weight (including battery):**   250 g

14. **Material in Case:**   plastic

15. **Material in Cover:**   clear plastic

16. **Special Features:**   Modes: DDD, DVI, VDD, DOO; AV delays: 10–250 msec, continuously adjustable. Transparent plastic cover to prevent unintentional control changes, capable of either unipolar or bipolar operation, flashing indicators (LED) for battery replacement, pulsing, and sensing.

17. **Price:** $5475

CARDIAC CONTROL SYSTEMS, INC.

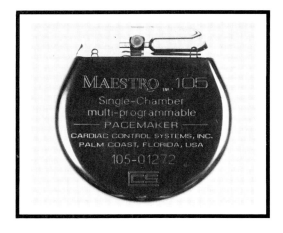 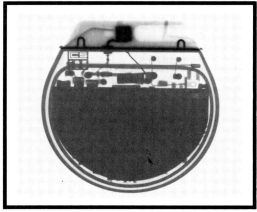

1. IDENTIFICATION/INFORMATION

Model:	105 Maestro (109 is similar)
24-Hr Telephone Number:	1-800-CCS-PACE (outside FL); 1-904-445-5450 (in FL)
Method of Operation (ICHD code):	VOO, VVI, VVT, AOO, AAI, AAT
Cost:	$4495 (1985)

2. SPECIAL FEATURES: compact lightweight, multiprogrammable, telemetry

3. PROGRAMMABLE FEATURES

Rate:	30 to 120 ppm (1-ppm steps)
Amplitude (voltage):	0.4, 0.8, 1.3, 1.7, 2.0, 2.5, 3.0, 3.5, 4.0, 5.0, 5.5, 6.0, "hi" V
Pulse Duration (width):	0.1 to 1.0 msec (0.1-msec steps)
Sensitivity:	1.4, 2.4, 2.8, 3.2, 4.5, 5.5 mV, low (L) and high (H) bandwidths for each value
Refractory:	100 to 600 msec (20-msec steps)
Changes of Mode (e.g., VVT to VVI):	VOO, VVI, VVT, AOO, AAI, AAT
Telemetry Response:	pacemaker series and programmed routine (mode + parameter values)
Other:	programmable only via Maestro model 1000 Pacemaker Programmer

4. ELECTRICAL CHARACTERISTICS

Sensitivity (mV):	as programmed
Pulse Duration (width):	as programmed
Pulse Amplitude (V):	as programmed
Energy (μjoules):	varies with programmed output and load
Basic Rate (ppm):	as programmed
Magnet Rate (ppm):	80
Refractory Period Pacing (msec):	as programmed
Refractory Period Sensing (msec):	as programmed (identical to above)
Escape Interval:	as programmed

5. POWER SOURCE

Number of Cells:	1
Manufacturer/Model Number:	WG 7911
Major Chemicals:	lithium iodine
Voltage (each cell):	2.8
Capacity:	2.5 amp-hr
Total Watt Hours:	6.75

6. LONGEVITY INFORMATION

Warranty:	8 yr
Manufacturer's Projected Life:	10.3 yr (100% pacing)

7. POWER SOURCE DEPLETION INDICATOR

Change in Pulse Rate:	change to 50 ppm at EOS
Change in Pulse Amplitude:	none
Other:	magnet rate modulation (70 to 80 ppm alternate beats) at ERI; magnet rate 50 ppm at EOS

8. METHOD FOR PERIODIC TEST OF PROPER FUNCTION

Magnet Test Rate:	80 ppm
Recommended Test Frequency:	4 to 6 wk; then every 3 mo
Does Magnet Work if Pacer Is Upside Down:	yes
Is Special Magnet Required:	no

9. EFFECT OF ELECTRICAL AND MAGNETIC FIELDS: reverts to fixed-rate pacing at programmed rate

10. PHYSICAL CHARACTERISTICS

Dimensions (mm):	$55 \times 51 \times 9$
Weight (g):	48
Volume (cc):	19.1
Materials in Contact With Tissue:	titanium, medical-grade epoxy, medical-grade silicone rubber
If Integral Part of Pulse Generator:	window in silicone rubber boot
Surface Area:	11.13 cm^2
Material:	titanium
Special Implant Position or Procedure:	no

11. NONINVASIVE IDENTIFICATION

X-ray Code (radiopaque letters):	CCS 105

12. TERMINAL CONNECTOR COMPATIBILITY

Cordis Lead:	with adapter
Medtronic Lead:	yes
Other:	all 5-mm lead connectors
Unipolar:	yes
Bipolar:	no
Both:	no
Accepts Atrial and Ventricular:	yes; one or the other

CARDIAC CONTROL SYSTEMS, INC.

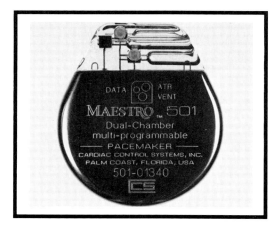 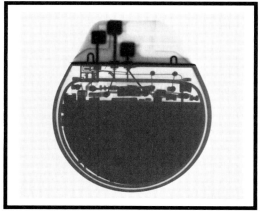

1. IDENTIFICATION/INFORMATION

Model:	501 (now in clinical trials)
24-Hr Telephone Number:	1-800-CCS-PACE (in FL 1-904-445-5450)
Method of Operation (ICHD code):	VOO, VVI, VVT, AOO, AAI, AAT, DOO, VDD, DVI, DDI, DDD-1, DDD-2, DDD-4
Cost:	$5795 (1985)

2. SPECIAL FEATURES: multiprogrammable, extensive telemetry including EGMs

3. PROGRAMMABLE FEATURES

Rate:	30 to 120 ppm (1-ppm steps)
Amplitude:	0.4, 0.8, 1.3, 1.7, 2.0, 2.5, 3.0, 3.5, 4.0, 5.0, 5.5, 6.0, ''HI'' V
Pulse Duration (width):	0.1 to 1.0 msec (0.1-msec steps)
Sensitivity:	0.5, 1.0, 1.4, 1.8, 2.4, 2.8, 3.2, 3.6, 4.5, 5.5, 6.4, 9.0, 11.0, 13.0, 18.0, 25.0 mV; low (L) and (H) bandwidths for each value
Refractory:	100 to 600 msec (20-msec steps)
Hysteresis:	
AV Delay:	60 to 300 msec (20-msec steps)
Changes of Mode (e.g., VVT to VVI):	VOO, VVI, VVT, AOO, AAI, AAT, DOO, VDD, DVI, DDI, DDD-1, DDD-2, DDD-3, DDD-4
Telemetry Response:	pacemaker series, programmed routine (mode and parameter values), system status data (cell voltage, elevated cell impedance warning, lead pacing currents, lead impedance); atrial and ventricular EGMs; dual-chamber capture EGM
Other:	programmed maximum AV follow rate mechanism precludes sustained PMT; time-limited AV capture test EGM and continuous AV EGM available when used with Polysafe model AV-102 AV Data Lead

4. ELECTRICAL CHARACTERISTICS

Sensitivity (mV):	as programmed
Pulse Duration (width):	as programmed
Pulse Amplitude (V):	as programmed
Energy (μjoules):	varies with programmed output and load
Current Consumption at 72 ppm 500 Ω (μamps):	
Current Consumption Inhibited (μamps):	
Basic Rate (ppm):	as programmed
Magnet Rate (ppm):	80

Refractory Period Pacing (msec):	as programmed
Refractory Period Sensing (msec):	as programmed (identical to above)
Escape Interval:	as programmed

5. POWER SOURCE

Number of Cells:	1
Manufacturer/Model Number:	WG 7911
Major Chemicals:	lithium iodine
Voltage:	2.8 V
Capacity:	2.5 amp-hr
Total Watt Hours:	6.75

6. LONGEVITY INFORMATION

Warranty:	4 yr
Manufacturer's Projected Life:	6.1 yr (100% pacing)

7. POWER SOURCE DEPLETION INDICATOR

Change in Pulse Rate:	change to 50 ppm at EOS
Change in Pulse Width:	none
Change in Pulse Amplitude:	none
Other:	magnet rate modulation (70 to 80 ppm alternate beats) at ERI; magnetic rate 50 ppm at EOS; telemetry warning printout

8. METHOD FOR PERIODIC TEST OF PROPER FUNCTION

Magnet Test Rate:	80 ppm
Recommended Test Frequency:	4 to 6 wk; then every 3 mo
Does Magnet Work if Pacer Is Upside Down:	yes
Is Special Magnet Required:	no

9. EFFECT OF ELECTRICAL AND MAGNETIC FIELDS: reverts to fixed-rate pacing at programmed rate

10. PHYSICAL CHARACTERISTICS

Dimensions (mm):	57 × 51 × 14
Weight (g):	65
Volume (cc):	33.8
Specific Gravity (g/cc):	
Material in Contact With Tissue:	titanium, medical-grade epoxy, medical-grade silicone rubber
Indifferent Electrode Characteristics if Integral Part of Pulse Generator:	window in silicone boot
Surface Area:	11.13 cm²
Material:	titanium
Special Implant Position or Procedure:	no

11. NONINVASIVE IDENTIFICATION

X-ray Code (radiopaque letters):	CCS 501
Other:	

12. TERMINAL CONNECTOR COMPATIBILITY

Cordis Lead:	with adapter
Medtronic Lead:	yes
Other:	A-V Data Lead™ all 5-mm lead connectors (connector plug provided if standard ventricular lead is used)
Unipolar:	yes
Bipolar:	no
Both:	no
Accepts Atrial and Ventricular:	yes; both simultaneously

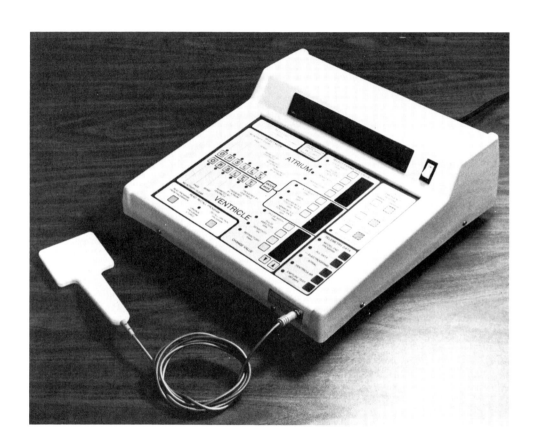

CARDIAC CONTROL SYSTEMS, INC.

1. IDENTIFICATION/INFORMATION
Model:	1000 Maestro Programmer

2. GENERAL DESCRIPTIONS
Pacemaker Models Programmed:	All Maestro series pacemakers
Power Source:	115 Vac
Fuse:	½ Amp AGC-type
Dimensions:	4⅞″ H × 15″ W × 15 ″ D
Weight:	11 lb
Method of Operation:	electronic transmission of biphase encoded information via programming wand
Operating Temperature:	ambient
Storage Temperature:	ambient

3. ACCESSORIES INFORMATION
Programming Wand and Cable Weight:	7.5 oz
Wand Cable Length:	6 ft
Power Cord Length:	7 ft

4. PROGRAMMING CAPABILITIES
Modes:	(depending on pacemaker model) VOO, VVI, VVT, AOO, AAI, AAT, DOO, VDD, DVI, DDI, DDD-1, DDD-2, DDD-3, DDD-4
Parameters:	(depending on pacemaker model) pacing rate, A-V delay, maximum A-V follow rate; atrial pulse width, pulse amplitude, sensitivity, refractory period; ventricular pulse width, pulse amplitude, sensitivity, refractory period
Telemetry Data:	(depending on pacemaker model) pacemaker series and programmed routine (mode and parameter values); time-limited atrial, ventricular, and capture test EGMs; continuous A-V EGM; system status data (cell voltage, elevated cell impedance warning, lead pacing currents, lead impedances)

5. SPECIAL FEATURES:
Switch on back of unit converts it to teaching tool for use in simulated programming experiences; pacing modes are entered via NASPE Specific Mode Code and are displayed in ICHD Generic Mode Code; wand is extremely lightweight and angled to facilitate use; alphanumeric display and human-engineered keyboard panel make device easy to use; provides for connection of Centronics-type printer and ECG recorder.

CARDIAC PACEMAKERS, INC.

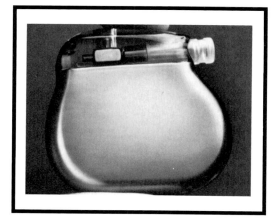 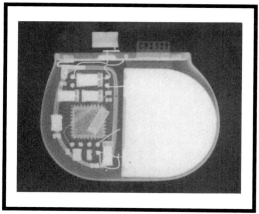

1. **IDENTIFICATION/INFORMATION**

Model:	ASTRA 6 429/529
24-Hr Telephone Number:	1-800-CARDIAC
Method of Operation (ICHD code):	VVI, AAI, VOO, AOO

2. **SPECIAL FEATURES:** stat 1 and 2 pacing modes; printout with 2035 programmer/printer

3. **PROGRAMMABLE FEATURES**

Rate:	prog: 30 to 120 ppm
Amplitude (current):	prog: 2.5, 5.0, 7.0
Pulse Duration (width):	prog: 0.03, 0.06, and 0.1 to 1.9 in 0.1-msec increments
Sensitivity:	prog: 0.5 to 3.0 in 0.5-mV increments and 5.0
Refractory:	prog: 250- to 500-msec increments
Changes of Mode (e.g., VVT to VVI):	see above
Telemetry Response:	all programmed values, plus stat 1 and 2, plus memory

4. **ELECTRICAL CHARACTERISTICS**

Sensitivity (mV):	see above
Pulse Duration (width):	see above
Pulse Amplitude (V):	prog: 2.5, 5.0, 7.0
Energy (μjoules):	22.5—factory setting
Current Consumption at 72 ppm:	19 μamps nominal (inhibited 9 μamps)
Basic Rate (ppm):	72
Magnet Rate (ppm):	100 BOL, single-step change to 87.5 at ERT
Pulse Interval Stability:	± 3 msec
Refractory Period Pacing (msec):	programmable
Refractory Period Sensing (msec):	250 to 500 msec in 25-msec increments

5. **POWER SOURCE**

Number of Cells:	1
Manufacturer/Model Number:	Wilson Greatbatch
Major Chemical:	lithium iodine
Voltage (each cell):	2.8
Capacity:	1.7 amp-hr

6. **LONGEVITY INFORMATION**

Warranty:	Pulse generator electrical components warranted for patient lifetime. Battery warranted for 8 years.

7. **POWER SOURCE DEPLETION INDICATOR**

Change in Pulse Rate:	12.5% single-step drop in programmed rate
Change in Pulse Width:	same as programmed

Change in Pulse Amplitude:	same as programmed
Other:	see *Telemetry*

8. METHOD FOR PERIODIC TEST OF PROPER FUNCTION

Magnet Test Rate:	100 ppm BOL
Other Changes:	none
Orientation of Magnet or Programmer When Being Applied to Pacer:	place over middle of PG parallel to lead connector
Does Magnet Work if Pacer Is Upside Down:	yes
Is Special Magnet Required:	standard CPI magnet 6511 for testing PG implanted less than 2.5 cm deep; large magnet CPI 6512 for testing PG implanted up to 4 cm deep

9. PHYSICAL CHARACTERISTICS

Weight (g):	48
Volume:	23 cc
Materials in Contact With Tissue:	hermetically sealed titanium
Indifferent Electrode Characteristic if Integral Part of Pulse Generator:	PG is coated with polymer leaving a small window of electrode area

10. NONINVASIVE IDENTIFICATION

X-ray Code (radiopaque letters):	CPI 529, CPI 629

11. TERMINAL CONNECTOR COMPATIBILITY

Unipolar:	529—5.38 mm = ''Cordis''
Bipolar:	429—3.2 mm ''in-line''
Accepts Atrial and Ventricular:	629—4.75 mm ''Medtronic''

12. TELEMETRY

: parameter status
: emergency STAT mode to nominal safety values
: programming completion signal
: pulse generator battery status
: 9-digit patient code
: connector size, lead type
: model and serial numbers

CARDIAC PACEMAKERS, INC.

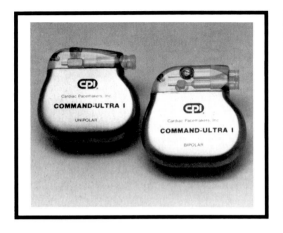
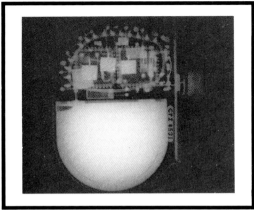

1. **IDENTIFICATION/INFORMATION**

Model:	Ultra I 531/631/635 (low profile)
24-Hr Telephone Number:	1-800-CARDIAC
Method of Operation (ICHD code):	VVI, AAI, VOO, AOO

2. **SPECIAL FEATURES:** Programmable and nonprogrammable memory, event counters, intra-cardiac electrogram. Printout with CPI 2031 printer. Restore mode.

3. **PROGRAMMABLE FEATURES**

Rate:	30 to 119 ppm
Amplitude (current):	2.5, 5.0, 7.5 V
Pulse Duration (width):	0.02 to 1.90 msec
Sensitivity:	off, 0.5 to 5.0 mV
Refractory:	250 to 400 msec
Hysteresis:	off, 50 to 400 msec
Changes of Mode (e.g. VVT to VVI):	VVI, AAI, VOO, AOO
Telemetry Response:	for all programmed values, EGM, memory
Other:	(memory is programmable)

4. **ELECTRICAL CHARACTERISTICS**

Sensitivity (mV):	see above
Pulse Duration (width):	see above
Pulse Amplitude (V):	see above
Energy (μjoules):	prog: .25 to 214
Current Consumption at 72 ppm, 500 Ω (μamps):	as programmed, 25 nominal
Current Consumption Inhibited (μamps):	13 nominal
Basic Rate (ppm):	prog: 30 to 119
Magnet Rate (ppm):	85 ppm
Pulse Interval Stability:	± 3 msec
Refractory Period Pacing (msec):	prog: 250 to 400 msec
Refractory Period Sensing (msec):	prog: 250 to 400 msec
Rate Hysteresis:	prog: 00 to 400 msec in 50-msec steps

5. **POWER SOURCE**

Manufacturer/Model Number:	Wilson Greatbatch
Major Chemical:	lithium iodine
Voltage (each cell):	2.8
Capacity:	1.7 amp-hr

6. **LONGEVITY INFORMATION**

Warranty:	pulse generator electrical components warranted for patient lifetime. Battery warranted for 8 years.

7. POWER SOURCE DEPLETION INDICATOR

Change in Pulse Rate:	−11%
Change in Pulse Width:	same as programmed
Change in Pulse Amplitude:	2.1 V when programmed to 2.5; 4.2 V when programmed to 5.0; 6.3 V when programmed to 7.5

8. METHOD FOR PERIODIC TEST OF PROPER FUNCTION

Magnet Test Rate:	100 ppm
Orientation of Magnet or Programmer When Being Applied to Pacer:	parallel to lead barrel, directly over PG

9. PHYSICAL CHARACTERISTICS

Dimensions (mm):	U—51 × 53 × 11 mm
	B—54 × 53 × 11 mm
	L/P—49 × 53 × 11 mm
Weight (g):	49, 49, 51, depending upon configuration
Volume (cc):	23
Materials in Contact With Tissue:	hermetically sealed titanium
Indifferent Electrode Characteristic if Integral Part of Pulse Generator:	unipolar PG is coated with polymer to decrease possibility of muscle stimulation, leaving a small window of electrode area.

10. NONINVASIVE IDENTIFICATION

X-ray Code (radiopaque letters):	CPI 531/631/635

11. TERMINAL CONNECTOR COMPATIBILITY

Cordis Lead:	531—5.38 mm = "Cordis"
Medtronic Lead:	631—4.75 = "Medtronic"
Other:	
Unipolar:	
Bipolar:	635—3.2 mm "in-line"
Both:	
Accepts Atrial and Ventricular:	

CARDIAC PACEMAKERS, INC.

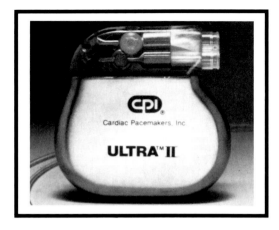
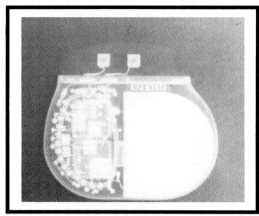

1. **IDENTIFICATION/INFORMATION**

Model:	Ultra II 910
24-Hr Telephone Number:	1-800-CARDIAC
Method of Operation (ICHD code):	VDD, VAT, VVI, VOO

2. **SPECIAL FEATURES:** Programmable and nonprogrammable memory, printout with CPI 2031 Printer, restore mode, atrial and ventricular intracardiac electrogram.

3. **PROGRAMMABLE FEATURES**

Rate:	prog: 30 to 90 ppm (LRL), prog: 100 to 180 (URL)
Amplitude (current):	2.5, 5.0, 7.5 V
Pulse Duration (width):	0.02 to 1.9 msec
Sensitivity:	A—off, 0.25 to 4.00 mV; V—off, 0.50 to 5.00 mV
Refractory:	A—175 to 475 msec (post-V); V—175 to 475 msec
AV Delay:	60 to 300 msec
Changes of mode (e.g., VVT to VVI):	VVD, VAT, VVI, VOO
Telemetry Response:	for all programmed values
Other:	EGM, memory

4. **ELECTRICAL CHARACTERISTICS**

Sensitivity (mV):	see above
Pulse Duration (width):	see above
Pulse Amplitude (V):	see above
Energy (μjoules):	prog: .25 to 214
Current Consumption at 72 ppm, 500 Ω (μamps):	as programmed, 25 nominal
Current Consumption Inhibited (μamps):	13 nominal
Basic Rate (ppm):	LRL—prog: 30 to 90 ppm
Magnet Rate (ppm):	100 ppm
Pulse Interval Stability:	± 3 msec
Refractory Period Pacing (msec):	see above
Refractory Period Sensing (msec):	see above

5. **POWER SOURCE**

Number of Cells:	1
Manufacturer/Model Number:	Wilson Greatbatch
Major Chemical:	lithium iodine
Voltage (each cell):	2.8
Capacity:	1.7 amp-hr

6. LONGEVITY INFORMATION

Warranty: Pulse generator electrical components warranted for patient lifetime. Battery warranted for 8 years.

7. POWER SOURCE DEPLETION INDICATOR

Change in Pulse Rate: -11%
Change in Pulse Width: same as programmed
Change in Pulse Amplitude: 2.1 V when prog. to 2.5, 4.2 V when prog. to 5.0, 6.0 V when prog. to 7.5

8. METHOD FOR PERIODIC TEST OF PROPER INDICATOR

Magnet Test Rate: 85 ppm
Orientation of Magnet or Programmer When Applied to Pacer: parallel to lead barrel, directly over PG

9. PHYSICAL CHARACTERISTICS

Dimensions (mm): 54 H $\times$ 53 W $\times$ 11 D
Weight (g): 51
Volume (cc): 25
Specific Gravity (g/cc): 2.04
Materials in Contact With Tissue: hermetically sealed titanium
Indifferent Electrode Characteristic if Integral Part of Pulse Generator: PG is coated with polymer to decrease possibility of muscle stimulation, leaving a small window of electrode area

10. NONINVASIVE IDENTIFICATION

X-ray Code (radiopaque letters): CPI 910

11. TERMINAL CONNECTOR COMPATIBILITY

Cordis Lead:
Medtronic Lead:
Other:
Unipolar: } 2 $\times$ 4.75 mm = "Medtronic"
Bipolar:
Both:
Accepts Atrial and Ventricular:

CARDIAC PACEMAKERS, INC.

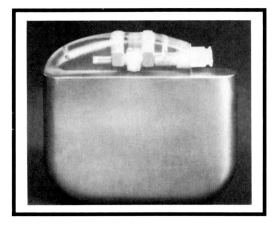
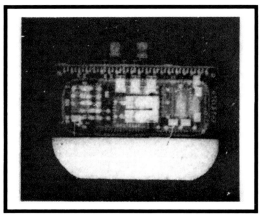

1. IDENTIFICATION/INFORMATION

Model:	Delta 925
24-Hr Telephone Number:	1-800-CARDIAC
Method of Operation (ICHD code):	DDD, VDD, DVI, DOO, AAI, AAT, AOO, VVI, VVT, VOO

2. SPECIAL FEATURES: rate smoothing, programmable fallback, programmable unipolar/bi-polar, stat 1 and 2 modes

3. PROGRAMMABLE FEATURES

Rate:	30 to 150 ppm
Amplitude (current):	2.2 to 8.2 V in 0.2-V increments
Pulse Duration (width):	A—0.05, 0.08, and 0.1 to 1.9 msec in 0.1-msec increments. V—0.05, 0.08, and 0.1 to 1.9 msec in 0.1-msec increments
Sensitivity:	(atrial) 0.25, 0.50, 0.75 mV and 1.0 to 10.0 mV in 0.5-mV increments, 11 to 15 mV in 1.0-mV increments (ventricular sens. see* below)
Refractory:	A (postV)—75 to 600 msec in 25-msec increments. V—75 to 600 msec in 25-msec increments
Hysteresis:	0 to 30 ppm below base rate in 1-ppm increments
AV Delay:	60 to 280 msec in 10-msec increments
Changes of Mode (e.g., VVT to VVI):	see above
Telemetry Response:	all programmed values

4. ELECTRICAL CHARACTERISTICS

Sensitivity (mV):	see above
Pulse Duration (width):	see above
Pulse Amplitude (V):	see above
Current Consumption at 72 ppm, 500 Ω (μamps):	as programmed, 58—2 chbr; 45—1 chbr
Current Consumption Inhibited (μamps):	32
Basic Rate (ppm):	prog: 30 to 150 ppm
Magnet Rate (ppm):	96—BOL, 85—ERT, gradual reduction from BOL to ERT
Pulse Interval Stability:	± 8 msec
Refractory Period Pacing (msec):	see above
Refractory Period Sensing (msec):	see above

---

* Ventricular Sensitivity: 0.25, 0.50, 0.75 V, 1.0 to 10.0 mV in 0.5-mV increments, 11 to 15 mV in 1.0-mV increments.

Rate Hysteresis:	prog: 0 to 30 ppm below base rate in 1-ppm increments

5. POWER SOURCE

Manufacturer/Model Number:	Wilson Greatbatch
Major Chemicals:	lithium iodine
Voltage (each cell):	2.8
Capacity:	2.35 amp-hr

6. LONGEVITY INFORMATION

Warranty:	pulse generator electrical components warranted for patient lifetime. Battery warranted for 6 years.

7. POWER SOURCE DEPLETION INDICATOR

Change in Pulse Rate:	same as programmed
Change in Pulse Width:	same as programmed

8. METHOD FOR PERIODIC TEST OF PROPER FUNCTION

Magnet Test Rate:	96 ppm—BOL, 85 ppm—ERT, gradual reduction from BOL to ERT
Does Magnet Work if Pacer Is Upside Down:	yes
Is Special Magnet Required:	no

9. PHYSICAL CHARACTERISTICS

Dimensions (mm):	56 H × 59 W × 12 D
Weight (g):	75
Volume (cc):	35
Materials in Contact With Tissues:	hermetically sealed titanium

10. NONINVASIVE IDENTIFICATION

X-ray Code (radiopaque letters):	CPI 0925

11. TERMINAL CONNECTOR COMPATIBILITY

Cordis Lead:
Medtronic Lead:
Other:
Unipolar:
Bipolar:
Both:
Accepts Atrial and Ventricular:

2 × 3.2 mm "in-line" = "Medtronic in-line"

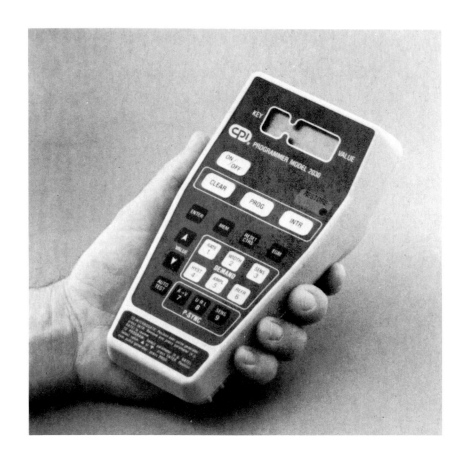

MANUFACTURER: Cardiac Pacemakers, Inc. (CPI)

MODEL: 2030 Programmer

1. **Carrier Frequency:**   40 kHz

2. **Data Bit Transmission Rate:**   250 kHz

3. **Programming Time (pulse period):**   Variable depending on parameter

4. **Programming Range:**   3.7 cm

5. **Display:**   4-digit LCD with decimal point, colons, and dashes

6. **Programmable Parameters**
   Rate: yes
   Hysteresis: yes
   Output: yes
   Pulse Width: yes
   Sensitivity: yes
   Mode: yes
   Refractory Period: yes
   Telemetry: yes
   Confirm Signal: yes—beeping
   Hard Copy Printer: used with Model 2031 printerbase

7. **Power Source:**   9-V battery

8. **Operating Time:**   12 hours continuous programming

9. **Pacemaker Series:**   Ultra I and II

10. **Dimensions:**   10.1 cm W × 19.3 cm L × 5.5 cm D

11. **Weight:**   492 g

12. **Special Features:**   EGM connector for intracardiac electrogram recording, real-time rate indication

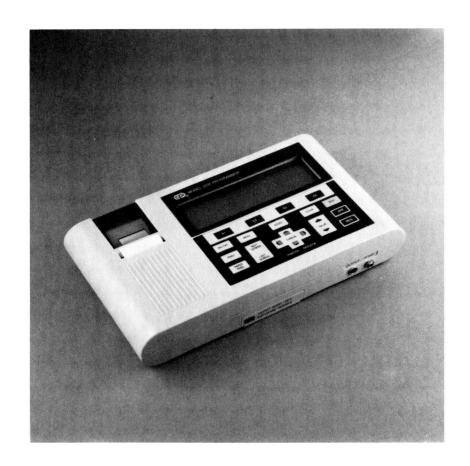

MANUFACTURER: Cardiac Pacemakers, Inc. (CPI)

MODEL: 2035 Hand-Held Programmer/Printer

1. **Carrier Frequency:**   100 kHz/40 kHz

2. **Data Bit Transmission Rate:**   1 kHz

3. **Programming Time (pulse period):**   0.5 to 2.0 sec

4. **Programming Range:**   1.5 inches

5. **Display:**   40 characters × 8 rows (320 characters) LCD

6. **Programmable Parameters**
   Rate: yes
   Output: yes
   Pulse Width: yes
   Sensitivity: yes
   Mode: yes
   Refractory Period: yes
   Telemetry: yes
   Hard Copy Printer: yes; uses 38-mm wide thermal printing paper

7. **Power Source:**   four 1.5-V AA batteries

8. **Operating Time:**   12 hours

9. **Pacemaker Series:**   Astra, Ultra, Delta

10. **Dimensions:**   15 cm W × 26.7 cm L × 4.5 cm H

11. **Weight:**   1150 g with plug-in module

12. **Special Features:**   The Model 2035 Programmer interrogates and programs different pulse generators, depending on the CPI software module selected.

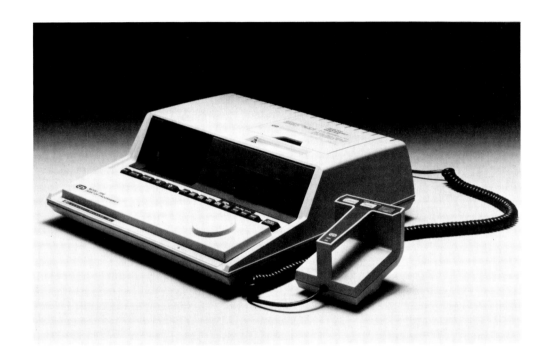

MANUFACTURER: Cardiac Pacemakers, Inc. (CPI)

MODEL: 2040 Programmer

1. **Carrier Frequency:**   100 kHz

2. **Data Bit Transmission Rate:**   1 kHz

3. **Programming Range:**   5 inches, used with telemetry wand with attached electronic module

4. **Display:**   video display screen

5. **Programmable Parameters**—determined by PG model
    Rate: 30 to 150 ppm
    Hysteresis: 30 ppm below base rate
    Output: 2.2 to 8.2 V, 0.2-V increments
    Pulse Width: 0.05, 0.08, 0.1 to 1.9 msec in 0.1-msec increments
    Sensitivity: .25, .50, .75 mV, 1.0 to 10.0 mV in 0.5-mV increments, 11 to 15 mV in 1.0-mV increments
    Mode: DDD, VDD, DVI, DOO, AAI, AAT, AOO, VVI, VVT, VOO
    Refractory Period: 75 to 600 msec in 25-msec increments
    Input Sensitivity: 15 mV
    Hard Copy Printer: Hewlett Packard paper 82954A—black, or Hewlett Packard 82931A—blue

7. **Power Source:**   115 V AC or 230 V AC, 50/60 Hz

8. **Power Consumption:**   40 Watts

9. **Operating Time:**   indefinite (line powered)

10. **Pacemaker Series:**   Delta (925)

11. **Dimensions:**   15 × 41.9 × 45.2 cm (6.3 × 16.5 × 17.8 in)

12. **Special Features:**   universal. Off-the-shelf device with plug-in modules. CRT, printer, key-entry in one unit.

CARDIO-PACE MEDICAL

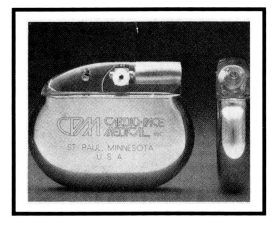 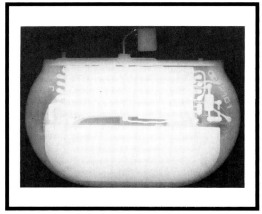

1. IDENTIFICATION/INFORMATION

Model:	Durapulse P101 Unipolar, P102 Bipolar
24-Hr Telephone Number:	1-612-483-6787 or 1-800-553-6036
Method of Operation (ICHD code):	VVI, VOO
Cost:	$1995

2. PROGRAMMABLE FEATURES

Rate:	programmable 30 to 120
Refractory:	programmable 310/405
Changes of Mode (e.g., VVT to VVI):	programmable VVI to VOO

3. ELECTRICAL CHARACTERISTICS

Sensitivity (mV):	± 2.2
Pulse Duration (width):	0.61 msec
Pulse Amplitude (V):	5.1 at pulse midpoint
Energy (μjoules):	32
Basic Rate (ppm):	programmable 30 to 120 ppm in 1-ppm increments
Magnet Rate (ppm):	same as programmed basic rate
Pulse Interval Stability:	crystal controlled
Refractory Period Pacing (msec):	310 or 405, programmable
Refractory Period Sensing (msec):	same as programmed refractory period pacing
Escape Interval:	500 msec to 2000 msec, programmable
Rate Hysteresis:	none

4. POWER SOURCE

Number of Cells:	1
Manufacturer/Model Number:	Wilson Greatbatch 7905
Configuration:	N/A
Major Chemicals:	lithium iodine
Voltage (each cell):	2.8
Capacity:	1.7 amp-hr
Total Watt Hours:	4.42 (based on 2.6 V)

5. LONGEVITY INFORMATION

Warranty:	5 years from date of implant
Manufacturer's Projected Life:	7.5 years at 50% pacing 750-ohm lead

6. POWER SOURCE DEPLETION INDICATOR

Change in Pulse Rate:	10% decrease

7. METHOD FOR PERIODIC TEST OF PROPER FUNCTION

Does Magnet Work if Pacer Is Upside Down:	yes
Is Special Magnet Required:	horseshoe magnet

8. PHYSICAL CHARACTERISTICS

Dimensions (mm):	45.6H × 56W × 11.5T (P101); 52H × 56W × 11.5T (P102)
Weight (g):	47 (P101), 51 (P102)
Volume (cc):	22 (P101), 25 (P102)
Specific Gravity (g/cc):	2.14 (P101), 2.04 (P102)
Materials in Contact With Tissue:	titanium, epoxy
If Integral Part of Pulse Generator:	pacemaker case (P101)
Material:	titanium
Special Implant Position/Procedure:	None

9. NONINVASIVE IDENTIFICATION

X-ray Code (radiopaque letters):	P101, P102

10. TERMINAL CONNECTOR COMPATIBILITY

Cordis Lead:	× (P101)
Medtronic Lead:	× (P102)

MANUFACTURER: Cardio-Pace Medical
MODEL: 1000 Programmer

1. **Carrier Frequency:**   262.5 kHz

2. **Data Bit Transmission Rate:**   128 Hz

3. **Programming Time (pulse period):**   86 msec

4. **Programming Range:**   1 inch

5. **Display:**   liquid crystal numeric

6. **Programmable Parameters**
    Rate: X
    Mode: X
    Refractory Period: X

7. **Power Source:**   9-V alkaline (Type 1604)

8. **Pacemaker Series:**   P101, P102

9. **Dimensions:**   14 cm L × 6.9 cm W × 3.7 cm T

10. **Weight:**   250 g

11. **Price:** $495

12. **Special Features:**   Test mode allows display of pulse generator rate as measured via skin electrodes on the patient.

CORDIS

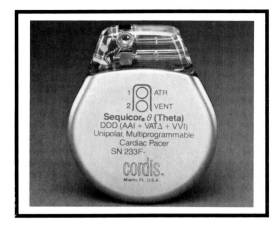 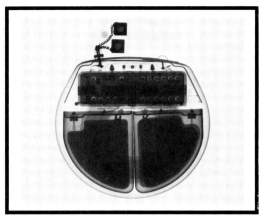

1. IDENTIFICATION/INFORMATION

Model:	Sequicor II, Model 233F
24-Hr Telephone Number:	1-800-327-8085 (outside FL); 1-800-432-6565 (within FL)
Method of Operation (ICHD code):	DDD, DAD, DVI, DOO, VDD, VAT, VVI, VOO
Cost:	$5295 (1984)

2. SPECIAL FEATURES: *Stat Set* (rapid programming to preselected values): VVI. 70 ppm, 1 msec, 10 mA, 1.3 mV

3. PROGRAMMABLE FEATURES

Rate:	30 to 120 ppm (in 5-ppm increments)

Amplitude and Pulse Duration Programmed in Combination

Amplitude Current:	2, 3, 4, 5, 6, 8, 10, 12 mA
Pulse Duration (width):	0.2, 0.3, 0.4, 0.5, 0.6, 0.8, 1.0, 2.0 msec
Sensitivity:	off, 0.5, 1.3, 2.5 mV (both channels, independent)
Refractory:	250, 300, 350, 400, 500 msec (both channels, independent)
AV Delay:	75, 100, 125, 150, 175, 200, 250 msec
Changes of Mode (e.g., VVT to VVI):	DDD, DAD, DVI, DOO, VDD, VAT, VVI, VOO
Telemetry Response:	programmed values
Other:	52½ ppm, VOO backup pacing

4. ELECTRICAL CHARACTERISTICS

Sensitivity (mV):	off, 0.5, 1.3, 2.5 (both channels, independent)
Pulse Duration (width):	0.2, 0.3, 0.4, 0.5, 0.6, 0.8, 1.0, 2.0 msec
Pulse Amplitude (V):	4.0, 8.4
Energy (μjoules):	14.4 nominal
Basic Rate (ppm):	70
Magnet Rate (ppm):	70
Pulse Interval Stability:	nonvariable
Refractory Period Pacing (msec):	250, 300, 350, 400, 500 (both channels, independent)
Refractory Period Sensing (msec):	250, 300, 350, 400, 500 (both channels, independent)
Escape Interval:	programmed rate

5. POWER SOURCE

Number of Cells:	2
Manufacturer/Model Number:	Cordis
Configuration:	approximately ¼ circular and in series

Major Chemicals:	lithium-cupric sulfide
Voltage (each cell):	2.1
Capacity:	2.1 amp-hr/cell
Total Watt Hours:	8.82

6. LONGEVITY INFORMATION

| Warranty: | prorated patient protection or replacement policy |
| Manufacturer's Projected Life: | 10 yr at 70 ppm, 0.6 msec/6 mA |

7. POWER SOURCE DEPLETION INDICATOR

| Change in Pulse Rate: | decrease to 62½ ppm (magnet applied) |

8. METHOD FOR PERIODIC TEST OF PROPER FUNCTION

Magnet Test Rate:	70 ppm
Other Changes:	Single Chamber—asynchronous
	Dual Chamber—atrial asynchronous ventricular inhibited during A-V delay
Recommended Test Frequency:	3-mo intervals
Orientation of Magnet or Programmer When Being Applied to Pacer:	within 1 in of reed switch
Does Magnet Work if Pacer Is Upside Down:	yes
Is Special Magnet Required:	no

9. EFFECT OF ELECTRICAL AND MAGNETIC FIELDS: See pacer *Instructions for Use*

10. PHYSICAL CHARACTERISTICS

Dimensions (mm):	69 × 57 × 15
Weight (g):	73
Volume (cc):	40.5
Specific Gravity (g/cc):	1.8
Material in Contact With Tissue:	titanium, epoxy, and silicone elastomer
Surface Areas:	61.5 cm^2
Material:	titanium
Special Implant Position/Procedure:	2 leads

11. NONINVASIVE IDENTIFICATION

| X-ray Code (radiopaque letters): | HK (233F) |

12. TERMINAL CONNECTOR COMPATIBILITY

Cordis Lead:	6-mm unipolar connectors
Medtronic Lead:	yes, with adapter
Other:	yes, with adapter
Unipolar:	yes
Bipolar:	no
Both:	no
Accepts Atrial and Ventricular:	yes, required

CORDIS

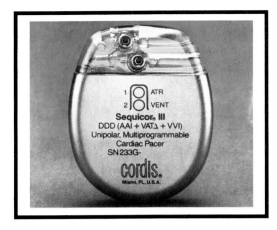 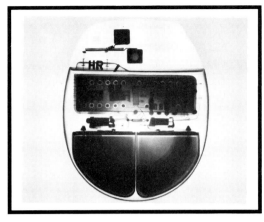

1. IDENTIFICATION/INFORMATION

Model: Sequicor III, Models 233G/GR/GL/GS

24-Hr Telephone Number: 1-800-327-8085 (outside FL); 1-800-432-6565 (within FL)

Method of Operation (ICHD code): DDD, DAD, DVI, DOO, VDD, VAT, VVI, VOO

Cost: $4995 (1985)

2. SPECIAL FEATURES: *Stat Set* (rapid programming to preselected values): VVI, 70 ppm, 1 msec, 10 mA, 1.3 mV

3. PROGRAMMABLE FEATURES

Rate: 30 to 120 ppm (in 5-ppm increments)

Amplitude and Pulse Duration Programmed in Combination

Amplitude (current): 2, 3, 4, 5, 6, 8, 10, 12 mA

Pulse Duration (width): 0.2, 0.3, 0.4, 0.5, 0.6, 0.8, 1.0, 2.0 msec

Sensitivity: off, 0.5, 1.3, 2.5 mV (both channels, independent)

Refractory: 250, 300, 350, 400, 500 msec (both channels, independent)

AV Delay: 75, 100, 125, 150, 175, 200, 250 msec

Changes of Mode (e.g., VVT to VVI): DDD, DAD, DVI, DOO, VDD, VAT, VVI, VOO

Telemetry Response: programmed values

Other: 52½ ppm, VOO backup pacing

4. ELECTRICAL CHARACTERISTICS

Sensitivity (mV): off, 0.5, 1.3, 2.5 (both channels, independent)

Pulse Duration (width): 0.2, 0.3, 0.4, 0.5, 0.6, 0.8, 1.0, 2.0 msec

Pulse Amplitude (V): 4.0, 8.4

Energy (μjoules): 14.4 nominal

Basic Rate (ppm): 70

Magnet Rate (ppm): 70

Pulse Interval Stability: nonvariable

Refractory Period Pacing (msec): 250, 300, 350, 400, 500 (both channels, independent)

Refractory Period Sensing (msec): 250, 300, 350, 400, 500 (both channels, independent)

Escape Interval: programmed rate

5. POWER SOURCE

Number of Cells: 2

Manufacturer/Model Number: Cordis

Configuration: approximately ¼ circular and in series

Major Chemicals:	lithium-cupric sulfide
Voltage (each cell):	2.1
Capacity:	0.88 amp-hr/cell (233G), 1.01 amp-hr/cell (233GL/GR/GS)
Total Watt Hours:	3.7 (233G), 4.24 (233GL/GR/GS)

6. LONGEVITY INFORMATION

| Warranty: | prorated patient protection or replacement policy |
| Manufacturer's Projected Life: | 5.0 yr at 70 ppm, 0.6 msec/6mA (233G); 5.8 yr at 70 ppm, 0.6 msec/6mA (233GR/GL) |

7. POWER SOURCE DEPLETION INDICATOR

| Change in Pulse Rate: | decrease to 62½ ppm (magnet applied) |

8. METHOD FOR PERIODIC TEST OF PROPER FUNCTION

Magnet Test Rate:	70 ppm
Other Changes:	single chamber—asynchronous; dual chamber—atrial asynchronous ventricular inhibited during A-V delay
Recommended Test Frequency:	3-mo intervals
Orientation of Magnet or Programmer When Being Applied to Pacer:	within 1 in of reed switch
Does Magnet Work if Pacer Is Upside Down:	yes
Is Special Magnet Required:	no

9. EFFECT OF ELECTRICAL AND MAGNETIC FIELDS: See pacer *Instructions for Use*

10. PHYSICAL CHARACTERISTICS

Dimensions (mm):	$57 \times 48 \times 10.4$
Weight (g):	43
Volume (cc):	23.8
Specific Gravity (g/cc):	1.8
Material in Contact With Tissue:	titanium, epoxy, and silicone elastomer
Surface Area:	28.4 cm^2
Material:	titanium
Special Implant Position/Procedure:	2 leads

11. NONINVASIVE IDENTIFICATION

| X-ray Code (radiopaque letters): | HR (233G), JP (233GL), JP (233GR), JP (233GS) |

12. TERMINAL CONNECTOR COMPATIBILITY

Cordis Lead:	4.75-mm unipolar (233G/GL), or 6-mm unipolar (233GR), or 3.2-mm unipolar (GS) connectors
Medtronic Lead:	yes, with adapter
Other:	yes, with adapter
Unipolar:	yes
Bipolar:	no
Both:	no
Accepts Atrial and Ventricular:	yes, required

CORDIS

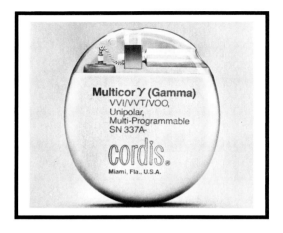

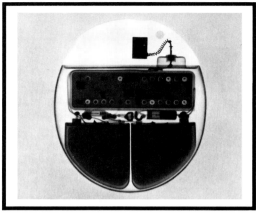

1. IDENTIFICATION/INFORMATION

Model: Multicor γ (Gamma), Models 336A/B and 337A

24-Hr Telephone Number: 1-800-327-8085 (outside FL); 1-800-432-6565 (within FL)

Method of Operation (ICHD code): VVI, VVT, VOO

Cost: $3550 Model 337A (1985); $3650 Model 336 A/B (1985)

2. SPECIAL FEATURES: *Stat Set* (rapid programming to preselected values): VVI, 70 ppm, 7 mA, 0.8 mV

3. PROGRAMMING FEATURES

Rate: 25 to 120 ppm

Amplitude (current): 1, 2, 4, 7 mA

Sensitivity: 0.8 to 5.5 mV

Refractory: 188 to 900 (rate dependent)

Changes of Mode (e.g., VVT to VVI): VVI, VVT, VOO

4. ELECTRICAL CHARACTERISTICS

Sensitivity (mV): 0.8 to 5.5

Pulse Duration (width): 1.25 msec

Pulse Amplitude (V): 4.1

Energy (μjoules): 5.3 to 36.8

Basic Rate (ppm): 70

Magnet Rate (ppm): same as programmed rate

Refractory Period Pacing (msec): 188 to 900 (rate dependent)

Escape Interval: programmed rate

5. POWER SOURCE

Number of Cells: 2

Manufacturer/Model Number: Cordis

Configuration: approximately ¼ circular and in series

Major Chemicals: lithium-cupric sulfide

Voltage (each cell): 2.1

Capacity: 0.88 amp-hr

Total Watt Hours: 3.69

6. LONGEVITY INFORMATION

Warranty: 7 yr

Manufacturer's Projected Life: 7 yr at 7 mA

7. POWER SOURCE DEPLETION INDICATOR

Change in Pulse Rate: 3% rate decrease

8. METHOD FOR PERIODIC TEST OF PROPER FUNCTION

Magnet Test Rate:	same as programmed rate
Recommended Test Frequency:	physician's discretion
Orientation of Magnet or Programmer When Being Applied to Pacer:	over reed switch and in center of pacer
Does Magnet Work if Pacer Is Upside Down:	yes
Is Special Magnet Required:	no

9. EFFECT OF ELECTRICAL AND MAGNETIC FIELDS: See pacer *Instructions for Use*

10. PHYSICAL CHARACTERISTICS

Dimensions (mm):	48 × 10 × 57
Weight (g):	41 (337A), 42 (336A/B)
Volume (cc):	18.6 (337A), 19.0 (336A/B)
Specific Gravity (g/cc):	2.2
Material in Contact With Tissue:	titanium, epoxy, and silicone elastomer
Surface Area:	27.36 cm^2
Material:	titanium

11. NONINVASIVE IDENTIFICATION

X-ray Code (radiopaque letters):	JD (337A), PX (336A/B)

12. TERMINAL CONNECTOR COMPATIBILITY

Cordis Lead:	yes, 336A (6-mm linear bipolar), 336B (4.75-mm bifurcated bipolar), 337A (6-mm unipolar)
Medtronic Lead:	yes, with adapters for 6-mm linear bipolar or unipolar
Other:	yes, with adapters
Unipolar:	yes
Bipolar:	yes (336A/B)
Both:	no
Accepts Atrial and Ventricular:	yes

CORDIS

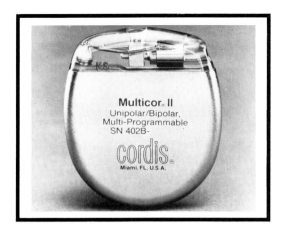 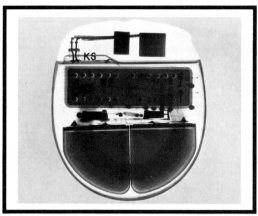

1. IDENTIFICATION/INFORMATION

Model:	Multicor II, Models 402A/B/C
24-Hr Telephone Number:	1-800-327-8085 (outside FL); 1-800-432-6565 (within FL)
Method of Operation (ICHD code):	VVI, VVT, VOO, VVI hysteresis, AAI, AAT, AOO
Cost:	$4295 (1985)

2. SPECIAL FEATURES: *Stat Set* (rapid programming to preselected values): VVI, 70 ppm, 7 mA, 1.3 mV

3. PROGRAMMABLE FEATURES

Rate:	off, 30 to 150 ppm (in 5-step increments)

Amplitude and Pulse Duration Programmed in Combination

Amplitude (current):	2, 3, 4, 5, 6, 8, 10, 12 mA
Pulse Duration (width):	0.2, 0.3, 0.4, 0.5, 0.6, 0.8, 1.0, 2.0 msec
Sensitivity:	0.5, 1.3, 2.5, 4.0 mV (VVI, VVT, AAI, AAT) 1.3, 2.0, 4.0 (VVI hysteresis only)
Refractory:	250, 300, 350, 400, 500 msec
Hysteresis:	0, 75, 100, 125, 150, 175, 200, 250 msec (VVI only)
Changes of Mode (e.g., VVT to VVI):	VVI, VVT, VOO, VVI hysteresis, AAI, AAT, AOO
Telemetry Response:	programmed values
Other:	polarity programmable; 52½ ppm, VOO backup pacing

4. ELECTRICAL CHARACTERISTICS

Sensitivity (mV):	0.5, 1.3, 2.5, 4.0 (VVI, VVT, AAI, AAT); 1.3, 2.0, 4.0 (VVI hysteresis only)
Pulse Duration (width):	0.2, 0.3, 0.4, 0.5, 0.6, 0.8, 1.0, 2.0 msec
Pulse Amplitude (V):	4.0, 8.4
Energy (μjoules):	14.4 nominal
Basic Rate (ppm):	70
Magnet Rate (ppm):	70
Pulse Interval Stability:	nonvariable
Refractory Period Pacing (msec):	250, 300, 350, 400, 500
Refractory Period Sensing (msec):	250, 300, 350, 400, 500
Escape Interval:	programmed rate

5. POWER SOURCE

Number of Cells:	2
Manufacturer/Model Number:	Cordis
Configuration:	approximately ¼ circular and in series
Major Chemicals:	lithium-cupric sulfide

Voltage (each cell):	2.1
Capacity:	0.88 amp-hr/cell
Total Watt Hours:	3.7

6. LONGEVITY INFORMATION

Warranty:	prorated patient protection or replacement policy
Manufacturer's Projected Life:	6.4 yr at 70 ppm, 0.6 msec/6 mA

7 POWER SOURCE DEPLETION INDICATOR

Change in Pulse Rate:	decrease to 62½ ppm (magnet applied)

8. METHOD FOR PERIODIC TEST OF PROPER FUNCTION

Magnet Test Rate:	70 ppm
Other Changes:	asynchronous
Recommended Test Frequency:	3-mo intervals
Orientation of Magnet or Programmer When Being Applied to Pacer:	within 1 in of reed switch
Does Magnet Work if Pacer Is Upside Down:	yes
Is Special Magnet Required:	no

9. EFFECT OF ELECTRICAL AND MAGNETIC FIELDS: See pacer *Instructions for Use*

10. PHYSICAL CHARACTERISTICS

Dimensions (mm):	57 × 48 × 10 (402A/B), 61 × 48 × 10 (402C)
Weight (g):	42
Volume (cc):	18.2
Specific Gravity (g/cc):	2.3
Material in Contact With Tissue:	titanium, epoxy, and silicone elastomer
Surface Area:	27.36 cm^2
Material:	titanium
Special Implant Position/Procedure:	402A (stencil side facing up)

11. NONINVASIVE IDENTIFICATION

X-ray Code (radiopaque letters):	HB (402A), KS (402B/C)

12. TERMINAL CONNECTOR COMPATIBILITY

Cordis Lead:	yes, 402A/B (6-mm unipolar or linear bipolar), 402C (4.75-mm bifurcated bipolar)
Medtronic Lead:	yes, with adapter
Other:	yes, with adapter
Unipolar:	yes
Bipolar:	yes, required for bipolar programming
Both:	yes
Accepts Atrial and Ventricular:	yes

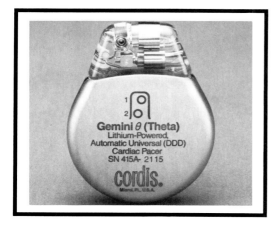 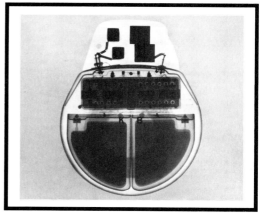

1. IDENTIFICATION/INFORMATION

Model:	Gemini θ (Theta), Model 415A
24-Hr Telephone Number:	1-800-327-8085 (outside FL); 1-800-432-6565 (within FL)
Method of Operation (ICHD code):	DDD, DVI, VDD, VVT, VVI, AAI, DDT/I, DDT, DAD, DVT, DAT, DOO, VOO, AOO
Cost:	$5750 (1985)

2. SPECIAL FEATURES: *Stat Set* (rapid programming to preselected values): VVI, 70 ppm, 1 msec, 10 mA, 1.3 mV

3. PROGRAMMABLE FEATURES

Rate:	off, 30 to 150 ppm (in 5-step increments)
Amplitude and Pulse Duration Programmed in Combination	
Amplitude (current):	2, 3, 4, 5, 6, 8, 10, 12 mA
Pulse Duration (width):	0.2, 0.3, 0.4, 0.5, 0.6, 0.8, 1.0, 2.0 msec
Sensitivity:	off, 0.5, 1.3, 2.5 mV (both channels, independent)
Refractory:	200, 250, 300, 350, 400, 500 msec (both channels, independent)
AV Delay:	0, 75, 100, 125, 150, 175, 200, 250 msec
Changes of Mode (e.g., VVT to VVI):	DDD, DVI, VDD, VVI, VVT, AAI, DDT/I, DDT, DAT, DVT, DAD, DOO, AOO, VOO
Telemetry Response:	programmed values
Other:	polarity programmable (VVI and VVT only) 52½ ppm, VOO backup pacing

4. ELECTRICAL CHARACTERISTICS

Sensitivity (mV):	off, 0.5, 1.3, 2.5 (both channels, independent)
Pulse Duration (width):	0.2, 0.3, 0.4, 0.5, 0.6, 0.8, 1.0, 2.0 msec
Pulse Amplitude (V):	4.0, 8.4
Energy (μjoules):	14.4 nominal
Basic Rate (ppm):	70
Magnet Rate (ppm):	70
Pulse Interval Stability:	nonvariable
Refractory Period Pacing (msec):	200, 250, 300, 350, 400, 500 (both channels, independent)
Refractory Period Sensing (msec):	200, 250, 300, 350, 400, 500 (both channels, independent)
Escape Interval:	programmed rate

5. POWER SOURCE

Number of Cells:	2
Manufacturer/Model Number:	Cordis

Configuration:	approximately ¼ circular and in series
Major Chemicals:	lithium-cupric sulfide
Voltage (each cell):	2.1
Capacity:	2.1 amp-hr/cell
Total Watt Hours:	8.82

6. LONGEVITY INFORMATION

| Warranty: | prorated patient protection or replacement policy |
| Manufacturer's Projected Life: | 10.0 yr at 70 ppm, 0.6 msec/6 mA |

7. POWER SOURCE DEPLETION INDICATOR

| Change in Pulse Rate: | decrease to 62½ ppm (magnet applied) |

8. METHOD FOR PERIODIC TEST OF PROPER FUNCTION

Magnet Test Rate:	70
Other Changes:	Single chamber—asynchronous Dual chamber—atrial asynchronous ventricular inhibited during A-V delay
Recommended Test Frequency:	3-mo intervals
Orientation of Magnet or Programmer When Being Applied to Pacer:	within 1 in of reed switch
Does Magnet Work if Pacer Is Upside Down:	yes
Is Special Magnet Required:	no

9. EFFECT OF ELECTRICAL AND MAGNETIC FIELDS: See pacer *Instructions for Use*

10. PHYSICAL CHARACTERISTICS

Dimensions (mm):	$57 \times 72 \times 15$
Weight (g):	73
Volume (cc):	40.5
Specific Gravity (g/cc):	1.8
Material in Contact With Tissue:	titanium, epoxy, and silicone elastomer
Surface Area:	61.5 cm^2
Material:	titanium
Special Implant Position/Procedure:	2 leads

11. NONINVASIVE IDENTIFICATION

| X-ray Code (radiopaque letters): | KB (415A) |

12. TERMINAL CONNECTOR COMPATIBILITY

Cordis Lead:	yes, 6-mm unipolar or linear bipolar connectors
Medtronic Lead:	yes, with adapters
Other:	yes, with adapters
Unipolar:	yes
Bipolar:	optional, linear bipolar ventricular only
Both:	no
Accepts Atrial and Ventricular:	yes, required

CORDIS

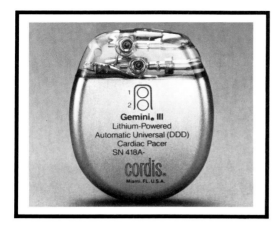
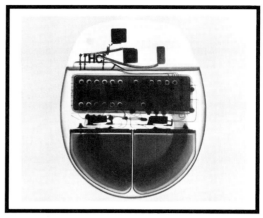

1. IDENTIFICATION/INFORMATION

Model:	Gemini III, Model 418A
24-Hr Telephone Number:	1-800-327-8085 (outside FL); 1-800-432-6565 (within FL)
Method of Operation (ICHD code):	DDD, DVI, VDD, VVI, VVT, AAI, DDT, DDT/I, DAD, DVT, DAT, DOO, VOO, AOO
Cost:	$5450 (1985)

2. SPECIAL FEATURES: *Stat Set* (rapid programming to preselected values): VVI, 70 ppm, 1 msec, 10 mA, 1.3 mV

3. PROGRAMMABLE FEATURES

Rate:	off, 30 to 150 ppm (in 5-ppm increments)

Amplitude and Pulse Duration Programmed in Combination

Amplitude (current):	2, 3, 4, 5, 6, 8, 10, 12 mA
Pulse Duration (width):	0.2, 0.3, 0.4, 0.5, 0.6, 0.8, 1.0, 2.0 msec
Sensitivity:	off, 0.5, 1.3, 2.5 mV (both channels, independent)
Refractory:	200, 250, 300, 350, 400, 500 msec (both channels, independent)
AV Delay:	0, 75, 100, 125, 150, 175, 200, 250 msec
Changes of Mode (e.g., VVT to VVI):	DDD, DVI, VDD, VVI, VVT, AAI, DDT/I, DDT, DAT, DVT, DAD, DOO, VOO, AOO
Telemetry Response:	programmed values
Other:	polarity programmable (VVI and VVT only) 52½ ppm, VOO backup pacing

4. ELECTRICAL CHARACTERISTICS

Sensitivity (mV):	off, 0.5, 1.3, 2.5 (both channels independent)
Pulse Duration (width):	0.2, 0.3, 0.4, 0.5, 0.6, 0.8, 1.0, 2.0 msec
Pulse Amplitude (V):	4.0, 8.4
Energy (μjoules):	14.4 nominal
Basic Rate (ppm):	70
Magnet Rate (ppm):	70
Pulse Interval Stability:	nonvariable
Refractory Period Pacing (msec):	200, 250, 300, 350, 400, 500 (both channels, independent)
Refractory Period Sensing (msec):	200, 250, 300, 350, 400, 500 (both channels, independent)
Escape Interval:	programmed rate

5. POWER SOURCE

Number of Cells:	2
Manufacturer/Model Number:	Cordis
Configuration:	approximately ¼ circular and in series

Major Chemicals:	lithium-cupric sulfide
Voltage (each cell):	2.1
Capacity:	1.01 amp-hr/cell
Total Watt Hours:	4.24

6. LONGEVITY INFORMATION

Warranty:	prorated patient protection or replacement policy
Manufacturer's Projected Life:	5.8 yr at 70 ppm, 0.6 msec/6 mA

7. POWER SOURCE DEPLETION INDICATOR

Change in Pulse Rate:	decrease to 62½ ppm (magnet applied)

8. METHOD FOR PERIODIC TEST OF PROPER FUNCTION

Magnet Test Rate:	70
Other Changes:	single chamber—asynchronous dual chamber—atrial asynchronous ventricular inhibited during A-V delay
Recommended Test Frequency:	3-mo intervals
Orientation of Magnet or Programmer When Being Applied to Pacer:	within 1 in of reed switch
Does Magnet Work if Pacer Is Upside Down:	yes
Is Special Magnet Required:	no

9. EFFECT OF ELECTRICAL AND MAGNETIC FIELDS: See pacer *Instructions for Use*

10. PHYSICAL CHARACTERISTICS

Dimensions (mm):	60 × 48 × 10.4
Weight (g):	43
Volume (cc):	23.8
Specific Gravity (g/cc):	2.2
Material in Contact With Tissue:	titanium, epoxy, and silicone elastomer
Surface Area:	28.45 cm²
Material:	titanium
Special Implant Position/Procedure:	2 leads

11. NONINVASIVE IDENTIFICATION

X-ray code (radiopaque letters):	HC (418A)

12. TERMINAL CONNECTOR COMPATIBLITY

Cordis Lead:	yes, 3.2-mm unipolar or linear bipolar connectors
Medtronic Lead:	yes, with adapters
Other:	yes, with adapters
Unipolar:	yes
Bipolar:	optional, linear bipolar ventricular only
Both:	no
Accepts Atrial and Ventricular:	yes, required

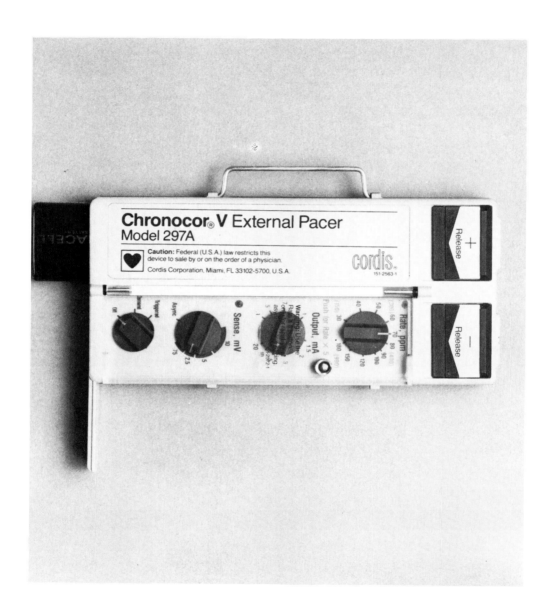

MANUFACTURER: Cordis Corporation

MODEL: 297A Chronocor V External Pacer

1. **Rate Range:**   30 to 180 ppm, 150 to 900 ppm (AOO only)

2. **Rate Calibration Accuracy:**   ± 10%

3. **Output Current Range:**   0.1 to 20 mA

4. **Current Calibration Accuracy:**   ± 10%

5. **Pulse Width:**   1.8 msec

6. **Sensitivity Range:**   0.75 to 10 mV

7. **Sensitivity Accuracy:**   ± 20%

8. **Refractory Period:**   325 msec

9. **Noise Rate (with EMI):**   reverts to VOO/AOO at set rate

10. **Power Source:**   9-V alkaline battery

11. **Battery Life:**   30 days at 60 ppm, 10 mA, and 100% pacing

12. **Physical Dimensions:**   12.7 cm × 6 cm × 2.2 cm

13. **Weight (including battery):**   190 g (8 oz)

14. **Material in Case:**   T-grade, ABS plastic

15. **Material in Cover:**   acrylic

16. **Special Features:**   Standard rate × 5 burst pulse for termination of supraventricular and re-entry tachycardias in atrium.

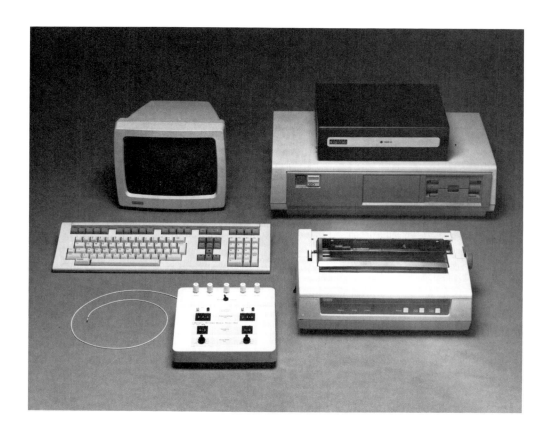

CORDIS

Cordis Computer-Driven, Dual-Channel Electrophysiology (EP) Stimulator

The Cordis Electrophysiology (EP) Stimulator is a software-based, computer-controlled system that uses the power of the DEC PC350 Professional Computer. Combined with specially designed EP software, the stimulator offers the physician a wide range of protocol programmability as well as the amenities associated with a personal computer.

FEATURES
1. The physician may design atrial, ventricular, or dual-channel protocols each tailored for a particular EP study.
2. A drive cycle is available within each protocol that may be used as a sensing drive, a pacing drive, or for burst pacing.
3. Four extrastimuli (S2 through S5) are available within each protocol at fully programmable intervals.
4. Automatic standby pacing is fully programmable in either atrial, ventricular, or dual-channel mode.
5. All protocols are synchronized to intrinsic events.
6. Single-channel protocols may be iterated, and all programmed intervals may be automatically increased or decreased between intervals.
7. Storage and instantaneous recall of up to four complete protocols.
8. All protocols used in a complete patient study are stored on disk for subsequent review.

TECHNICAL DATA

Number of Drive Cycles:	0 to 100
Drive Cycle (S_1–S_1) Interval:	140 to 1000 msec
Drive Cycle Interval Ramp:	-100 to 100 msec
S_1–S_2 Interval:	140 to 1000 msec
S_2–S_3 Interval:	140 to 1000 msec
S_3–S_4 Interval:	140 to 1000 msec
S_4–S_5 Interval:	140 to 1000 msec
Number of Iterations:	1 to 100
Automatic Increment/Decrement Applicable to Drive Cycle and Extrastimuli Intervals:	-100 to 100 msec
Channel 1 to Channel 2 Delay:	-250 to 250 msec

STANDBY PACING PARAMETERS

Pacing Intervals:	500 to 2000 msec
A-V Delay:	20 to 300 msec
Atrial Refractory:	400 to 600 msec
Ventricular Refractory:	250 to 600 msec

OUTPUT

Pulse Duration:	off, 0.1 to 4 msec
Pulse Amplitude:	0.2 to 29.9 mA
Sensitivity:	off, 0.5 to 7.5 mV
Power Source*:	120 VAC (isolated)
Recommended Operating Conditions:	10° to 40°C (50° to 104°F), 20 to 80% relative humidity

---

* A 120 VAC Isolation Transformer is supplied with each system.

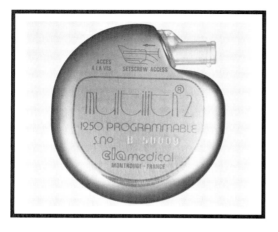
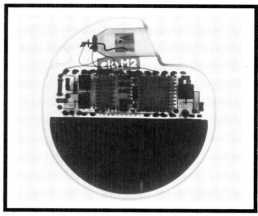

1. IDENTIFICATION/INFORMATION

Model:	Multilith 2 1250 Monopolar; 2250 Bipolar
Method of Operation (ICHD code):	VVI M

2. PROGRAMMABLE FEATURES

Rate:	30 to 50 to 120 cpm (by 5 cpm)
Amplitude (current):	2.5, 5, 7.5 V
Sensitivity:	1 to 2 to 3 to 4 mV
Refractory:	310 to 470 msec
Changes of Mode (e.g., VVT to VVI):	VOO, VVI, VVT
Telemetry Response:	all parameters
Other:	threshold test—magnet rate

3. ELECTRICAL CHARACTERISTICS

Sensitivity (mV):	1, 2, 3, 4
Pulse Duration (width):	0.5 msec
Pulse Amplitude (V):	2.5, 5, 7.5
Energy (μjoules):	24
Current Consumption at 72 ppm 500 Ω (μamps):	22
Current Consumption Inhibited (μA):	9.5
Basic Rate (ppm):	70
Magnet Rate (ppm):	86
Pulse Interval Stability:	3 msec
Refractory Period Pacing (msec):	310
Refractory Period Sensing (msec):	290
Escape Interval:	pacing period

4. POWER SOURCE

Number of Cells:	1
Manufacturer/Model Number:	WG 8077
Major Chemicals:	LiI_2
Voltage (each cell):	2.8
Capacity:	1.8
Total Watt Hours:	5

5. LONGEVITY INFORMATION

Manufacturer's Projected Life:	8.5 yr (under normal values)

6. POWER SOURCE DEPLETION INDICATOR:

Magnetic Pulse Rate:	86 to 77 cpm (1 step)

7. METHOD FOR PERIODIC TEST OF PROPER FUNCTION

Magnet Test Rate:	86 cpm
Orientation of Magnet or Programmer When Being Applied to Pacer:	1 PM

Does Magnet Work if Pacer Is Upside Down: yes
Is Special Magnet Required: no

8. EFFECTS OF ELECTRICAL AND MAGNETIC FIELDS: VOO

9. PHYSICAL CHARACTERISTICS

Dimensions (mm): $50 \times 54 \times 9.4$
Weight (g):   47
Volume (cc):   20
Specific Gravity (g/cc):   2.35
Materials in Contact With Tissue: pure titanium
Surface Area: 45 cm^2
Material: titanium
Special Implant Position/Procedure: no

10. NONINVASIVE IDENTIFICATION

X-ray Code (radiopaque letters):   ELA M2

11. TERMINAL CONNECTOR COMPATIBILITY

Cordis Lead: no
Medtronic Lead: yes
Unipolar: Model 1250
Bipolar: Model 2250
Both: no
Accepts Atrial and Ventricular: no

ELA MEDICAL

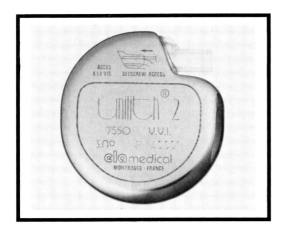 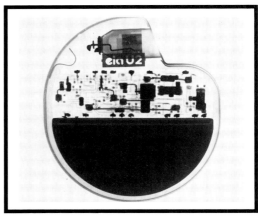

1. **IDENTIFICATION/INFORMATION**

Model:	Unilith 2 (7550)
Method of Operation (ICHD code):	VVI

2. **PROGRAMMABLE FEATURES:** none

3. **ELECTRICAL CHARACTERISTICS**

Sensitivity (mV):	2
Pulse Duration (width):	0.5 msec (7550), 0.7 msec (7760)
Pulse Amplitude (V):	5
Energy (μjoules):	22 (7550), 28 (7760)
Current Consumption at 72 ppm, 500 Ω (μamps):	17.5
Current Consumption Inhibited (μA):	5.5
Basic Rate (ppm):	70
Magnet Rate (ppm):	70
Pulse Interval Stability:	3 msec
Refractory Period Pacing (msec):	310
Refractory Period Sensing (msec):	310
Escape Interval:	pacing period

4. **POWER SOURCE**

Number of Cells:	1
Manufacturer/Model Number:	WG 8077 (7550), CRC 910 (7660)
Major Chemicals:	LiI
Voltage (each cell):	2.8
Capacity:	1.6 (7550), 1.5 (7760)
Total Watt Hours:	4.46 (7750), 4.20 (7760)

5. **LONGEVITY INFORMATION**

Manufacturer's Projected Life:	11 yr (7550), 7 yr (7660)

6. **POWER SOURCE DEPLETION INDICATOR**

Change in Pulse Rate:	−4 ppm
Change in Pulse Width:	+0.02 msec
Change in Pulse Amplitude:	−1 V

7. **METHOD FOR PERIODIC TEST OF PROPER FUNCTION**

Magnet Test Rate:	70 ppm
Recommended Test Frequency:	1 year
Orientation of Magnet or Programmer When Being Applied to Pacer:	1 PM
Does Magnet Work if Pacer Is Upside Down:	yes
Is Special Magnet Required:	no

8. **EFFECTS OF ELECTRICAL AND MAGNETIC FIELDS:** VOO

9. PHYSICAL CHARACTERISTICS

Dimensions (mm):	$54 \times 50 \times 8.4$
Weight (g):	41
Volume (cc):	18
Material in Contact With Tissue:	pure titanium
Material:	titanium

10. NONINVASIVE IDENTIFICATION

X-ray Code (radiopaque letters):	ELA U2

11. TERMINAL CONNECTOR COMPATIBILITY

Cordis Lead:	no
Medtronic Lead:	yes

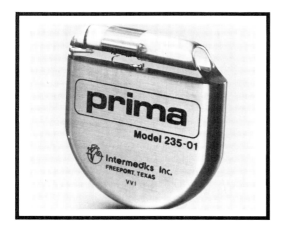 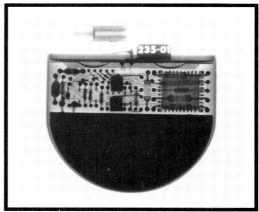

1. **IDENTIFICATION/INFORMATION**

Model:	Prima 235-01
24-Hr Telephone Number:	1-800-231-2330; in Texas 1-800-392-3726
Method of Operation (ICHD code):	VVI
Cost:	$2295 (1985)

2. **SPECIAL FEATURES:** Intermedics Inter-Lock connector

3. **PROGRAMMABLE FEATURES:** Not programmable

4. **ELECTRICAL CHARACTERISTICS**

Sensitivity (mV):	2.4
Pulse Duration (width):	0.49 to 0.52 msec
Pulse Amplitude (V):	not less than 5.2
Basic Rate (ppm):	72 ± 2
Magnet Rate (ppm):	nominally, same as beginning of service stim- ulation rate
Refractory Period:	316 ± 24 msec
Upper Rate Limit:	135 ppm

5. **POWER SOURCE**

Number of Cells:	1
Manufacturer/Model Number:	WGL 8077
Major Chemicals:	lithium iodine
Voltage:	2.8
Capacity:	1.8 amp-hr

6. **POWER SOURCE DEPLETION INDICATOR**

Change in Pulse Rate:	a magnet mode pacing rate of 66 ± 4 ppm

7. **METHOD FOR PERIODIC TEST OF PROPER FUNCTION**

Magnet Test Rate:	yes

8. **EFFECT OF ELECTRICAL AND MAGNETIC FIELDS:** reverts to VOO pacing at 88 ± 7 ppm

9. **PHYSICAL CHARACTERISTICS**

Dimensions (mm):	50 × 47 × 8
Weight (g)	40
Material in Contact With Tissue	titanium with conformal polymer coating, bi- ologically compatible epoxy, medical grade silicone rubber, acetal polymer

10. **NONINVASIVE IDENTIFICATION**

X-ray Code (radiopaque letters):	235-01

11. TERMINAL CONNECTOR COMPATIBILITY*: accepts leads with standard 6-mm connectors

---

* Model 236-02 accepts bifurcated bipolar 5-mm leads

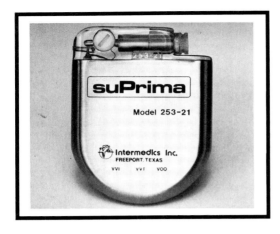
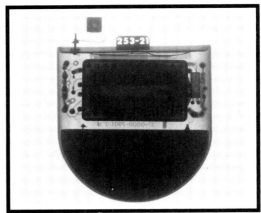

1. **IDENTIFICATION/INFORMATION**

Model:	SuPrima 253-21
24-Hr Telephone Number:	1-800-231-2330; in Texas 1-800-392-3726
Method of Operation (ICHD code):	VVI, VVT, VOO
Cost:	$2995 (1985)

2. **SPECIAL FEATURES:** program confirmation

3. **PROGRAMMABLE FEATURES**

Rate:	30, 40, 50, 60, 66, 69, 72, 76, 80, 85, 90, 96, 103, 111, 120 ppm
Pulse Duration (width):	0.15, 0.31, 0.46, 0.61, 0.76, 0.92, 1.07, 1.22, 1.37, 1.53, 1.68, 1.83, 1.98, 2.14, 2.29 msec
Amplitude:	9.76 mA (at leading edge with 500 ohms)
Sensitivity:	1.0 to 4.6 mV (7 settings)
Changes of Mode (e.g., VVT to VVI):	VVI, VVT, VOO
Telemetry Response:	programming confirmation

4. **OTHER ELECTRICAL CHARACTERISTICS**

Basic Rate (ppm):	72
Magnet Rate (ppm):	90
Refractory Period:	332 msec (290 for rates 111 and 120)
Upper Rate Limit:	125.7 ppm

5. **POWER SOURCE**

Number of Cells:	1
Manufacturer/Model Number:	WG 8074
Major Chemicals:	lithium iodine
Voltage:	2.8
Capacity:	2 to 3 amp-hr
Total Watt Hours:	6.21

6. **POWER SOURCE DEPLETION INDICATOR**

Change in Pulse Rate:	7 ppm decrease in magnet rate from BOS rate
Change in Pulse Amplitude:	not less than 3.6 V at leading edge

7. **METHOD FOR PERIODIC TEST OF PROPER FUNCTION**

Magnet Test Rate:	yes

8. **EFFECT OF ELECTRICAL AND MAGNETIC FIELDS:** VVI mode: reverts to VOO at 90 ppm; VVT mode: paces synchronously to a maximum of 125.7 ppm

9. **PHYSICAL CHARACTERISTICS**

Dimensions (mm):	60 × 47 × 11
Weight (g):	60

Material in Contact With Tissue: titanium, polymer coating, silicone, acetyl polymer

10. NONINVASIVE IDENTIFICATION
X-ray Code (radiopaque letters):   253-21 on connector

11. TERMINAL CONNECTOR COMPATIBILITY*
Cordis Lead: yes
Medtronic Lead: with adapter
Unipolar: yes

---

* Model 254-12 5-mm bifurcated bipolar; Model 254-24 6-mm in-line bipolar

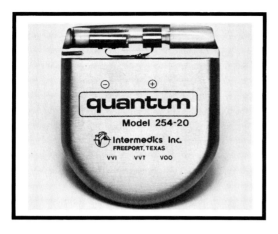
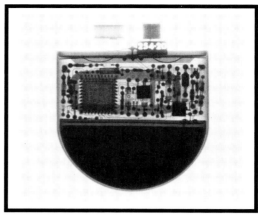

1. IDENTIFICATION/INFORMATION

Model:	Quantum 254-20*
24-Hr Telephone Number:	1-800-231-2330; in Texas 1-800-392-3726
Method of Operation (ICHD code):	VVI, VVT, VOO
Cost:	$4395 (1985)

2. SPECIAL FEATURES: see 12. Telemetry; Model 253-19 accepts *bifurcated* bipolar connections

3. PROGRAMMABLE FEATURES

Rate:	30, 40, 50, 60, 69, 72, 76, 80, 85, 90, 96, 103, 111, 120
Amplitude:	2.7, 5.4, 8.1 V
Pulse Duration (width):	0.15, 0.31, 0.46, 0.61, 0.76, 0.92, 1.07, 1.22, 1.37, 1.53, 1.68, 1.83, 1.98, 2.14, 2.29 msec
Sensitivity:	0.6, 1.2, 1.8, 2.4, 3.0, 3.6, 4.2 mV
Changes of Mode (e.g., VVT to VVI):	VVI, VVT, VOO
Telemetry:	on (transmission terminates automatically after 15 sense or pace events)

4. OTHER ELECTRICAL CHARACTERISTICS

Pulse Amplitude (V):	(BOL) 5.4, (EOL) 4.2
Magnet Rate (ppm):	(BOL) 87 ± 3, (EOL) 80 ± 2
Refractory Period:	322 msec (rates 30 to 103); 290 msec (rates 111 or 120)
Upper Rate Limit:	125

5. POWER SOURCE

Number of Cells:	1
Manufacturer/Model Number:	CRC 910 or WG 8077
Major Chemicals:	lithium iodine
Voltage:	2.8
Capacity:	1.8 amp-hr

6. POWER SOURCE DEPLETION INDICATOR

Change in Magnet Rate:	goes from 87 ± 3 (BOL) to 80 ± 2 ppm
Available via Telemetry:	A decline in power cell voltage to 2.2 V (magnet mode) at EOL.

7. METHOD FOR PERIODIC TEST OF PROPER FUNCTION

Magnet Test Rate:	see 6 above

8. EFFECT OF ELECTRICAL AND MAGNETIC FIELDS: VVI mode: reverts to VOO at 90 ppm; VVT mode: paces synchronously to a maximum of 125.7 ppm

---

* 253-09* unipolar; 254-09* bipolar, 5-mm bifurcated; 254-10* bipolar, Intermedics in-line connector; 253-19 unipolar; 254-18 bipolar, 5-mm bifurcated; 254-20 bipolar, Intermedics in-line connector

9. **PHYSICAL CHARACTERISTICS**

Dimensions (mm):	54 × 47 × 8
Weight (g):	41
Material in Contact With Tissue:	titanium with conformal polymer coating, medical grade silicone rubber, biologically compatible epoxy and acetal polymer

10. **NONINVASIVE IDENTIFICATION**

X-ray Code (radiopaque numbers):	254-20

11. **TERMINAL CONNECTOR COMPATIBILITY:** accepts Intermedics in-line bipolar leads having 6-mm connectors

12. **TELEMETRY:** (programmed telemetry, magnet telemetry) rate, interval, pulse width, pulse amplitude, output pulse current, lead impedance, charge delivered, energy delivered, power cell voltage, average power cell current, power cell impedance

INTERMEDICS

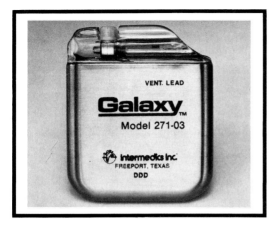 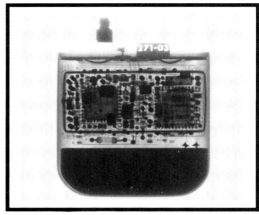

1. IDENTIFICATION/INFORMATION

Model:	Galaxy 271-03
24-Hr Telephone Number:	1-800-231-2330; in Texas 1-800-392-3726
Method of Operation (ICHD code):	DDD
Cost:	$5195 (1985)

2. SPECIAL FEATURES: see 11. Telemetry and diagnostic data; see 6. Replacement indicator

3. PROGRAMMABLE FEATURES

Rate:	30 to 120 ppm in 1-ppm increments
Amplitude:	A: 2.7, 5.4, 8.1 V; V: 2.7, 5.4, 8.1 V
Pulse Duration (width):	A: 0.03 to 1.5 msec by 0.01 steps; V: 0.03 to 1.5 msec by 0.01 steps
Sensitivity:	A: 0.4, 0.8, 1.2, 1.6, 2.0, 2.4, 2.8 mV; V: 1.0, 2.0, 3.0, 4.0, 5.0, 6.0, 7.0 mV
Refractory:	A: (Total) 220 to 570 msec in 5-msec increments; (PVARP) 170 to 520 msec in 5-msec increments; V: 170 to 320 msec in 5-msec increments
AV Delay:	50 to 300 msec in 5-msec increments
Changes of Mode (e.g., VVT to VVI):	DDD, VDD, DVI, DVI(C), DOO, VVI, VVT, VOO, AAI, AAT, AOO
Ventricular Tracking Limit (VDD and DDD modes):	94 to 100 ppm in 2-ppm increments
Special Programmable Adjustments:	15.5 to 75 msec in 2.5-msec increments
Telemetry Response:	see 11 below

4. ELECTRICAL CHARACTERISTICS

BOS Output Current:	10.8 mA into 500 ohms at 0.45 msec
Magnet Rate:	asynchronous pacing at programmed parameters
Atrial Refractory Extension:	100 msec
Nonphysiologic AV Delay:	100 msec
Run Away; Upper Rate Limit:	185 ppm

5. POWER SOURCE

Number of Cells:	1
Manufacturer/Model Number:	WG 7905
Major Chemicals:	lithium iodine
Voltage:	2.8
Capacity:	1.7 amp-hr

6. POWER SOURCE DEPLETION INDICATOR

Intensified Follow-up Indicator:	reversion to single-chamber asynchronous pacing at 90 ppm in magnet mode

Elective Replacement Indicator: reversion to single-chamber pacing at pro-grammed parameters in the nonmagnet mode. Reversion to single-chamber asyn-chronous pacing at 80 ppm in the magnet mode

7. METHOD FOR PERIODIC TEST OF PROPER FUNCTION
Magnet Test Rate: yes

8. PHYSICAL CHARACTERISTICS
Dimensions (mm): 58 × 47 × 11
Weight (g): 55
Material in Contact With Tissue: titanium with polymer coating, biologically compatible epoxy, medical grade silicone rub-ber, acetal polymer

9. NONINVASIVE IDENTIFICATION
X-ray Code (radiopaque letters): 271-03

10. TERMINAL CONNECTOR COMPATIBILITY: accepts 2 unipolar leads with 5-mm connectors

11. TELEMETRY: *Inquire data* (programmed parameters): Pulse generator serial number, mode, rate, pacing interval, A-V delay, refractory periods (A & V), ventricular tracking limit, maximum pacing rate, pulse width, pulse amplitude, sensitivity; *Diagnostic data* (a record of categorized pacing/sensing variables documenting pacemaker-patient interaction): Number of times: tracking limit reached, PMT termination algorithm activated; Number of: premature V events, A sense events followed by a V sense event, A sense event followed by a V pace event, A pace events followed by a V pace event, V sense events not preceded by an A pace event, V pace events not preceded by an A sense event, A sense events, A pace events, V sense events, V pace events

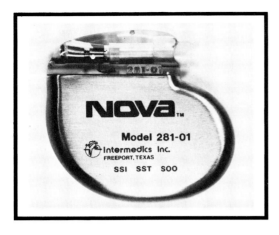 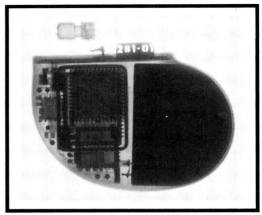

1. IDENTIFICATION/INFORMATION

Model:	Nova 281-01
24-Hr Telephone Number:	1-800-231-2330; in Texas 1-800-392-3726
Method of Operation (ICHD code):	SSI, SST, SOO, OOO
Cost:	$4595 (1985)

2. SPECIAL FEATURES

Telemetry:	measured values and diagnostic data. Threshold margin test

3. PROGRAMMABLE FEATURES

Rate:	30 to 120 ppm in 1-ppm increments
Amplitude:	2.7, 5.4, 3.1 V
Pulse Duration (width):	0.03 to 1.5 msec in 0.01-msec increments
Sensitivity:	1.0, 2.0, 3.0, 4.0, 5.0, 6.0, 7.0 mV
Refractory:	170 to 400 msec in 5-msec increments
Hysteresis:	30 to 120 bpm in 1-bpm increments
Changes of Mode:	SSI, SST, SOO, OOO
Telemetry Response:	see 12 below

4. OTHER ELECTRICAL CHARACTERISTICS

Magnet Rate (ppm):	90 ppm for 4 cycles, then SOO at programmed rate
Upper Rate Limit:	185 ppm

5. POWER SOURCE

Number of Cells:	1
Manufacturer/Model Number:	WGL 8041
Major Chemicals:	lithium iodine
Voltage:	2.8
Capacity:	2.2 amp-hr

6. POWER SOURCE DEPLETION INDICATOR

- Reversion to pacing at 65 ppm in the programmed mode (except SST mode changes to SSI mode)

7. METHOD FOR PERIODIC TEST OF PROPER FUNCTION

Threshold Margin Test:	at beginning of 5th output cycle following induction of magnet mode, pulse width is reduced by one half; loss of capture indicates that pulse width may need to be increased

8. EFFECT OF ELECTRICAL AND MAGNETIC FIELDS: above 7 events/sec reverts to VOO pacing at programmed rate.

9. PHYSICAL CHARACTERISTICS

Dimensions (mm):	54 × 51 × 10
Weight (g):	49
Case:	titanium
Seal:	hermetic
Header:	biologically compatible epoxy
Suture Hole Plug:	medical-grade silicone rubber
Screw Cap:	acetal polymer
Material in Contact With Tissue:	titanium with a conformal polymer coating, biologically compatible epoxy, medical grade silicone rubber, acetal polymer

10. NONINVASIVE IDENTIFICATION

X-ray Code (radiopaque letters):	281-01 on connector

11. TERMINAL CONNECTOR COMPATIBILITY:* accepts standard 6-mm connectors

Unipolar:	yes

12. TELEMETRY

Inquire:	all programmed settings plus model and serial numbers
Measured Values:	(accuracy)
Pacing Rate:	± 2.0 ppm
Pacing Interval:	± 1.5%
Pulse Width:	± 0.01 msec
Pulse Amplitude:	± 10%
Output Current:	± 15%
Load Impedance:	± 15%
Charge Delivered:	± 15%
Energy Delivered:	± 20%
Power Cell Voltage:	± 10%
Power Cell Impedance:	± 1 KΩ or ± 15%, whichever is greater
Diagnostic Data (in SSI mode):	date counter last cleared, number of pace events, number of sense events, percent paced

---

* Model 282-02 accepts an Intermedics 6-mm in-line bipolar lead.

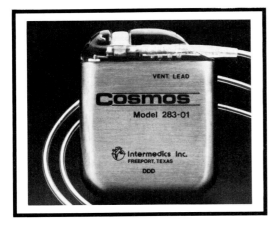
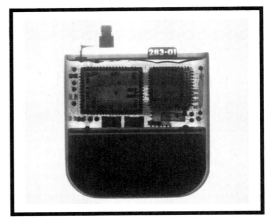
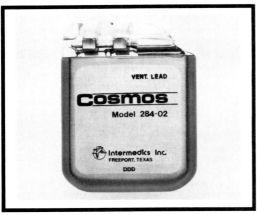
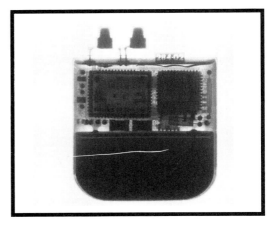

1. **IDENTIFICATION/INFORMATION**

Model:	Cosmos 283-01 (unipolar)*; Cosmos 284-02 (bipolar)
24-Hr Telephone Number:	1-800-231-2330; in Texas 1-800-392-3726
Method of Operation (ICHD code):	DDD
Cost:	$5895

2. **SPECIAL FEATURES:** critical pacing functions are programmable in smaller increments; advanced telemetry (see 11 below); threshold margin test

3. **PROGRAMMABLE FEATURES**

Rate:	30 to 120 ppm in 1-ppm increments
Amplitude:	A: 2.7, 5.4, 8.1 volts; V: 2.7, 5.4, 8.1 volts
Pulse Duration (width):	A: 0.03 to 1.5 msec in 0.01-msec steps; V: 0.03 to 1.5 msec in 0.01-msec steps
Sensitivity:	A: 0.4 to 2.8 by 0.4-mV steps; V: 1.0 to 7.0 by 1.0-mV steps
Refractory:	A: 220 to 570 by 5-msec steps; V: 170 to 320 by 5-msec steps
AV Delay:	50 to 300 by 5-msec steps
Change of Mode:	DDD, VDD, DVI (C), DVI, DOO, VVI, VVT, VOO, AAI, AAT, AOO, OOO (off)
Ventricular Tracking Limit (VDD and DDD modes):	94 to 180 ppm in 2-ppm increments

---

* 284-01 is similar except it accepts two Intermedics in-line bipolar leads

Atrial Refractory Extension:	0 to 250 msec in 5-msec increments
Fallback Deceleration:	2.5 to 100 msec per pulse in 2.5-msec increments
Ventricular Blanking Period:	15.5 to 75 msec in 2.5-msec increments
Nonphysiologic A-V Delay:	50 to 160 msec in 5-msec increments
Deactivation of Elective Replacement Indicator:	on/off
Hysteresis (minimal unpaced rate VVI and AAI modes):	30 to 120 bpm in 1-bpm increments

4. OTHER ELECTRICAL CHARACTERISTICS

Magnet Rate (ppm):	90 ppm for 4 cycles, then asynchronous at programmed
Upper Rate Limit:	185

5. POWER SOURCE

Number of Cells:	1
Major Chemicals:	lithium iodine
Voltage:	2.8
Capacity:	3.0 amp-hr
Total Watt Hours:	7.8

6. POWER SOURCE DEPLETION INDICATOR

Change in Pulse Rate:	to VVI at 65 ppm

7. METHOD FOR PERIODIC TEST OF PROPER FUNCTION

Magnet Test Rate:	yes
Threshold Margin Test:	at beginning of 5th output cycle following induction of magnet mode, pulse width is reduced by one half; loss of capture indicates that pulse width may need to be increased

8. PHYSICAL CHARACTERISTICS

Dimensions (mm):	$60 \times 47 \times 11$
Weight (g):	65

9. NONINVASIVE IDENTIFICATION

X-ray Code (radiopaque numbers):	283-01

10. TERMINAL CONNECTOR COMPATIBILITY

Dual Unipolar:	accepts two unipolar leads with standard 5-mm connectors

11. TELEMETRY

- Inquire data (programmed parameters)
- Telemetry data (measured pacing, lead system and battery parameters)
- Diagnostic data (a record of 10 categorized pacing/sensing variables documenting pacer-patient interaction, stored in pacer memory and retrievable by interrogation)

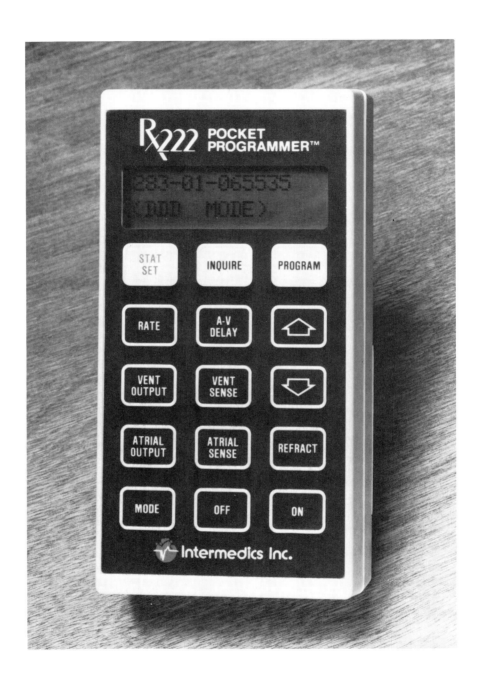

MANUFACTURER: Intermedics, Inc.

MODEL: 320-02 "Pocket Programmer"

1. **Carrier Frequency:**   N/A (pulse position–modulated signal)

2. **Data Bit Transmission Rate:**   2 pulses per 1/1024 second (average)

3. **Programming Time (pulse period):**   approximately 4 seconds depending on pacemaker model being programmed and the amount of environmental electrical interference

4. **Programming Range:**   1½ in (minimum) from pulse generator

5. **Display:**   liquid crystal dot matrix

6. **Programmable Parameters**
   Rate: yes
   Hysteresis: yes
   Output: yes
   Pulse Width: yes
   Sensitivity: yes
   Mode: yes
   Refractory Period: yes
   Confirm Signal: yes
   Input Sensitivity: yes
   Hard Copy Printer: no

7. **Power Source:**   standard 9-V alkaline battery

8. **Power Consumption:**   N/A

9. **Operating Time:**   approximately 5 hours, continuous

10. **Pacemaker Series:**   271-03, 281-01, 282-02, 283-01, 284-02

11. **Dimensions:**   15.3 × 7.8 × 2.8 cm (6.0 × 3.1 × 1.1 in)

12. **Weight:**   280 g (10 oz)

13. **Special Features:**

   • Small size, light weight; conveniently fits in shirt pocket
   • Large, 2-line character display for programming, inquire data, and operating instructions

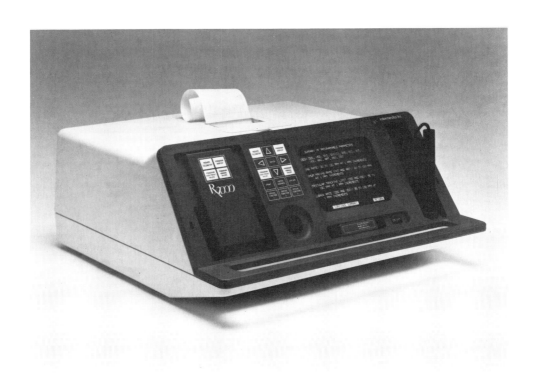

MANUFACTURER: Intermedics, Inc.

MODEL: 522-06 Programmer

1. **Carrier Frequency:**   N/A (pulse position–modulated signal)

2. **Data Bit Transmission Rate:**   2 pulses per 1/1024 second (average)

3. **Programming Time (pulse period):**   40 msec to 210 msec depending on pacemaker model being programmed, and amount of environmental electrical interference

4. **Programming Range:**   1½ in from pulse generator

5. **Display:**   CRT (6-in diagonal) display of programming, telemetry data, and operating information

6. **Programmable Parameters:**   All parameters for Intermedics programmable pulse generators

   Rate: yes
   Hysteresis: yes
   Output: yes
   Pulse Width: yes
   Sensitivity: yes
   Mode: yes
   Refractory Period: yes
   Confirm Signal: yes
   Input Sensitivity: yes
   Hard Copy Printer: yes

7. **Power Source:**   110 V: 95–130V, 45–65 Hz, a.c.; 220 V: 190–260 V, 45–65 Hz, a.c.

8. **Power Consumption:**   75 Watts

9. **Operating Time:**   N/A (line powered)

10. **Pacemaker Series:**   251, 252, 253, 254, 259, 262, 271, 281, 282, 283, 284

11. **Dimensions:**   43.8 × 44.2 × 21.6 cm (17¼ × 17⅜ × 8½ in)

12. **Weight:**   25 lb

13. **Special Features:**

   • Light pen for quick selection of functions from CRT display "menus"
   • Plug-in "program modules" for updating capabilities as new pacemaker models and operating features are introduced
   • Large CRT screen displays programming and telemetry information as well as operating instructions and "explain" screen

MEDTRONIC, INC.

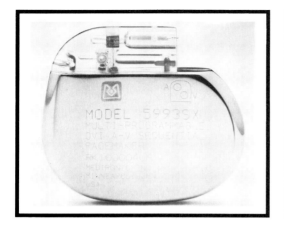 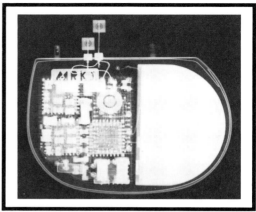

1. IDENTIFICATION/INFORMATION

Model:	Byrel-SX, Model 5993-SX
24-Hr Telephone Number:	1-800-328-2518
Method of Operation (ICHD code):	DVI,M
Cost:	$4500 (1984)

2. SPECIAL FEATURES: ventricular safety pacing

3. PROGRAMMABLE FEATURES

Rate:	40 to 120 ppm (DVI); 40 to 130 ppm (VVI) for the lower rate
Amplitude (voltage):	4.85
Pulse Duration (width):	0.05, .1 to 1.5 msec (steps of .1 msec), atrial and ventricular
Sensitivity:	2.5, 5.0 mV and asynchronous (ventricular)
Refractory:	235 msec (ventricular)
Hysteresis:	not available
AV Delay:	25 to 250 msec (steps of 25 msec)
Changes of Mode:	DVI, VVI, and asynchronous
Telemetry Response:	not available
Other:	ventricular safety pacing (110 msec AV interval)

4. ELECTRICAL CHARACTERISTICS

Sensitivity:	measured at a 10-msec sine^2 waveform
Pulse Duration (width):	± 7%
Pulse Amplitude (V):	4.6 minimum
Energy (μjoules):	varies with programmed pulse widths
Current Consumption:	varies with programmed pulse width
Basic Rate (ppm):	programmable
Magnet Rate (ppm):	same as programmed (DVI and VVI)
Pulse Interval Stability:	± 2 ppm
Refractory Period Pacing (msec):	235
Refractory Period Sensing (msec):	235
Escape Interval:	same as programmed
Rate Hysteresis:	none

5. POWER SOURCE

Number of Cells:	1
Manufacturer/Model Number:	Promeon/Beta 263
Voltage (each cell):	2.8
Capacity:	2.6 amp-hr (available); 1.95 amp-hr deliverable

6. LONGEVITY INFORMATION

Warranty:	limited warranty for 4 yr

7. **POWER SOURCE DEPLETION INDICATOR**

Change in Pulse Rate:	in DVI, 75 ppm at stage 1 and 65 ppm at stage 2 (elective replacement)
Change in Pulse Width:	automatic increase to maintain a nearly constant energy per pulse, as amplitude decreases
Change in Pulse Amplitude:	proportional to power source voltage decrease
Other:	reverts to VVI at stage 2

8. **METHODS FOR PERIODIC TEST OF PROPER FUNCTION**

Magnet Test Rate:	same as programmed
Other Changes:	threshold margin test, with three paired pulses 10% faster than magnet rate, with the pulse widths of the third pulses reduced by 25%
Recommended Test Frequency:	physician option
Orientation of Magnet or Programmer When Applied to Pacer:	against skin, over and parallel to the pacemaker
Does Magnet Work if Pacer Is Upside Down:	yes
Is Special Magnet Required:	yes, though programming head suffices

9. **EFFECT OF ELECTRICAL AND MAGNETIC FIELDS:** depending on the signal's strength, the unit may continue sensing, revert to asynchronous operation, or trigger synchronized ventricular pacing

10. **PHYSICAL CHARACTERISTICS**

Dimensions (mm):	52 (H) × 60 (L) × 10 (T)
Weight (g):	52
Volume (cc):	23
Materials in Contact With Tissue:	titanium, polyurethane, silicone rubber
Part of Pulse Generator:	elliptical window in the external coating
Surface Area:	approximately 2 in^2
Material:	titanium
Special Implant Position or Procedure:	uncoated side to face toward skin

11. **NONINVASIVE IDENTIFICATION**

X-ray Code (radiopaque letters):	RK
Others:	first symbol is Medtronic logo; the number after the letter is the engineering series number

12. **TERMINAL CONNECTOR COMPATIBILITY**

Cordis Lead:	some leads, without adapters
Medtronic Lead:	yes
Other:	with adapters
Accepts Atrial and Ventricular:	note that these leads must be inserted into the proper lead ports for dual-chamber pacing to occur

MEDTRONIC, INC.

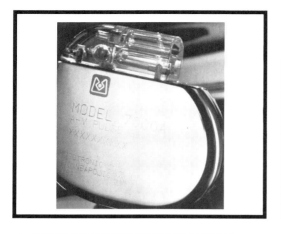 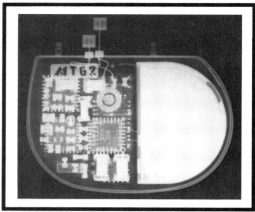

1. **IDENTIFICATION/INFORMATION**

Model:	Versatrax II, Model 7000A
24-Hr Telephone Number:	1-800-329-2518
Method of Operation (ICHD code):	DDD, M
Cost:	$4800 (1984)

2. **SPECIAL FEATURES:** automatic atrial refractory extension, ventricular safety pacing

3. **PROGRAMMABLE FEATURES**

Rate:	40 to 80 ppm (DDD); 40 to 120 ppm (DVI); 40 to 130 ppm (VVI) for the lower rate; upper rates are 100, 125, 150, and 175 ppm
Amplitude (voltage):	4.85
Pulse Duration (width):	0.05, .1 to 1.5 msec (steps of .1 msec) for both atrial and ventricular
Sensitivity:	0.75, 1.5, 3.0 mV and asynchronous (atrial); 2.5, 5.0 mV and asynchronous (ventricular)
Refractory:	235 (both atrial and ventricular); both extend to 340 msec automatically after a PVC
Hysteresis:	not available
AV Delay:	25 to 250 msec (steps of 25 msec)
Changes of Mode:	DDD, DVI, VVI, and asynchronous
Telemetry Response:	not available
Other:	ventricular safety pacing (110 msec AV interval)

4. **ELECTRICAL CHARACTERISTICS**

Sensitivity:	atrial: at a 10-msec sine^2 waveform, and ventricular: at a 40-msec sine^2 waveform
Pulse Duration (width):	± 7%
Pulse Amplitude (V):	4.6 minimum
Energy (μjoules):	varies with programmed pulse widths
Current Consumption:	varies with programmed pulse width
Basic Rate (ppm):	programmable
Magnet Rate (ppm):	85 ppm (DDD); as programmed (DVI and VVI)
Pulse Interval Stability:	± 2 ppm
Refractory Period Pacing (msec):	235
Refractory Period Sensing (msec):	235, but atrial and ventricular extend to 340 after a PVC
Escape Interval:	same as programmed
Rate Hysteresis:	none

5. POWER SOURCE

Number of Cells:	1
Manufacturer/Model Number:	Promeon/Beta 263
Voltage (each cell):	2.8
Capacity:	2.6 amp-hr (available); 1.95 amp-hr deliverable

6. LONGEVITY INFORMATION

Warranty:	limited warranty for 4 yr

7. POWER SOURCE DEPLETION INDICATION

Change in Pulse Rate:	in DDD, 75 ppm at stage 1 and 65 ppm at stage 2 (elective replacement)
Change in Pulse Width:	automatic increase to maintain a nearly constant energy per pulse, as amplitude decreases
Change in Pulse Amplitude:	proportional to decrease in power source voltage
Other:	reverts to VVI at stage 2

8. METHOD FOR PERIODIC TEST OF PROPER FUNCTION

Magnet Test Rate:	85 ppm in the DDD mode
Other Changes:	threshold margin test, with three paired pulses 10% faster than magnet rate, with the pulse widths of the third pulses reduced by 25%
Recommended Test Frequency:	physician option
Orientation of Magnet or Programmer When Applied to Pacer:	against skin, over and parallel to the pulse generator
Does Magnet Work if Pacer Is Upside Down:	yes
Is Special Magnet Required:	yes, though programming head suffices

9. EFFECT OF ELECTRICAL AND MAGNETIC FIELDS: depending on the signal's strength, the unit may continue sensing, revert to asynchronous operation, or trigger synchronized ventricular pacing

10. PHYSICAL CHARACTERISTICS

Dimensions (mm):	52 (H) $\times$ 60 (L) $\times$ 10 (T)
Weight (g):	52
Volume (cc):	23
Materials in Contact With Tissue:	titanium, polyurethane, silicone rubber
Indifferent Electrode Characteristic if Integral Part of Pulse Generator:	elliptical window in the external coating
Surface Area:	approximately 2 in^2
Material:	titanium
Special Implant Position/Procedure:	uncoated side to face toward skin

11. NONINVASIVE IDENTIFICATION

X-ray Code (radiopaque letters):	TG
Other:	first symbol is Medtronic logo; the number after the letter is the engineering series number

12. TERMINAL CONNECTOR COMPATIBILITY

Cordis Lead:	some leads, without adapters
Medtronic Lead:	yes
Other:	with adapters
Accepts Atrial and Ventricular:	note that these leads must be inserted into the proper lead ports for dual-chamber pacing to occur

MEDTRONIC, INC.

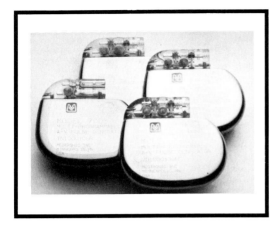 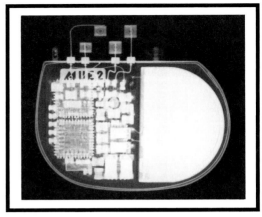

1. IDENTIFICATION/INFORMATION

Model: Symbios 7005 dual unipolar, 7005C dual universal unipolar, 7006 dual bipolar

24-Hr Telephone Number: 612-328-2518

Method of Operation (ICHD code): DDD, C

Cost: $5500 (7005/05C), $5600 (7006)—1985

2. SPECIAL FEATURES: all three models are A-V universal pacemakers, equipped with telemetry, marker channel, EGM, automatic atrial refractory extension, and tachycardia report

3. PROGRAMMABLE FEATURES

Rate: 40 to 130 ppm (in steps of 10 ppm) for the lower rate; upper rate is programmable from 100 to 175 ppm (in steps of 25 ppm); 135 to 400 ppm (temporary, in steps of 10/20 ppm)

Amplitude (current): 2.5 or 5.0 V

Pulse Duration (width): 0.05 to 1.5 msec (steps of 0.05 up to .8 msec and then .1-msec steps thereafter)

Sensitivity: 0.6, 1.25, 2.5, 5.0 mV and asynchronous (ventricular)

Refractory: 155, 225, 325, 400 (atrial); 225 (ventricular)—automatic extension to 400 msec and 345 msec, respectively, after a PVC (DDD mode only)

AV Delay: 25 to 250 msec (steps of 25)

Changes of Mode: DDD, DVI, VVI, AOO, DOO, VOO

Telemetry Response: pacemaker ID; status of programmable parameters; battery status; marker channel, and EGM

Other: ventricular safety pacing, temporary programming of some parameters

4. ELECTRICAL CHARACTERISTICS

Sensitivity: atrial: at a 10-msec sine^2 waveform, and ventricular: at a 40-msec sine^2 waveform

Pulse Duration (width): from .05 to .25 msec, the tolerance is $\pm$ 30% and from .3 to 1.5 msec, it is $\pm$ 7%

Pulse Amplitude (V): the minimum amplitude for the 2.5-V setting is 2.1, and for the 5.0-V setting it is 4.6

Energy (μjoules): depends on programmed settings

Basic Rate (ppm): programmable

Magnet Rate (ppm): 85 (DDD)

Pulse Interval Stability: $\pm$ 2 ppm

Refractory Period Pacing (msec): atrial: programmable to 155, 225, 325, 400 ($+10$ and -20 msec)

Refractory Period Sensing (msec): as above, but automatically extends after a PVC in the DDD mode only to 400 (atrial) and 345 (ventricular)

Escape Interval:	same as programmed basic rate and/or magnet rate
Rate Hysteresis:	none

5. POWER SOURCE

Number of Cells:	1
Manufacturer/Model Number:	Promeon/Beta 263
Major Chemicals:	lithium iodine
Voltage (each cell):	2.8
Capacity:	2.6 amp-hr (max available capacity), with 2.0 amp-hr deliverable

6. LONGEVITY INFORMATION

Warranty:	lifetime limited warranty on components and workmanship, battery warranted for 10 yr with full replacement for battery failure up to 4 yr for 7005 and 7005C, and 5 yr for 7006, and prorated for the remainder

7. POWER SOURCE DEPLETION INDICATOR

Change in Pulse Rate:	in DDD mode, to 75 ppm at stage 1 and to 65 ppm at stage 2
Change in Pulse Width:	automatic increase to maintain a nearly constant energy per pulse, as amplitude decreases
Other:	reverts to VVI at stage 2; telemetry reports both stages

8. METHOD FOR PERIODIC TEST OF PROPER FUNCTION

Magnet Test Rate:	85 ppm in DDD mode
Other Changes:	threshold margin test, with 3 pulses 10% faster than magnet rate, with the width of the third pulse reduced by 25%
Recommended Test Frequency:	physician option
Orientation of Magnet or Programmer When Applied to Pacer:	against skin, over and parallel to generator
Does Magnet Work if Pacer Is Upside Down:	yes
Is Special Magnet Required:	yes, though programming head suffices

9. EFFECT OF ELECTRICAL AND MAGNETIC FIELDS: the bipolar model has virtually eliminated sensing of EMI and myopotentials. The unipolar model may, depending on the signal's intensity, continue sensing, revert to asynchronous operation, or trigger synchronized ventricular pacing

10. PHYSICAL CHARACTERISTICS

Dimensions (mm):	52 (H) × 60 (L) × 10 (T)
Weight (g):	51 (7005); 53 (7006)
Volume (cc):	23
Materials in Contact With Tissue:	titanium, polyurethane, silicone rubber
Indifferent Electrode Characteristic if Integral Part of Pulse Generator:	elliptical window in external coating on the Models 7005 and 7005C
Surface Area:	approximately 2 in² (Models 7005 and 7005C)
Material:	titanium
Special Implant Position/Procedure:	no special position for the Model 7006, but with Models 7005 and 7005C, the uncoated side must face toward skin

11. NONINVASIVE IDENTIFICATION

X-ray Code (radiopaque letters):	7005: TN, 7005C: JS, 7006: UE
Other:	first symbol is Medtronic logo; the number after the letters is the engineering series number

12. TERMINAL CONNECTOR COMPATIBILITY

Cordis Lead:	yes (Model 7005C)
Medtronic Lead:	yes
Other:	with adapters
Accepts Atrial and Ventricular:	note that these leads must be inserted into the proper lead ports for dual-chamber pacing to occur

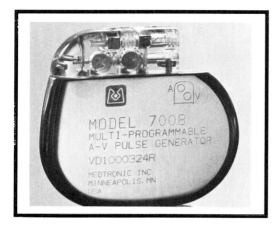
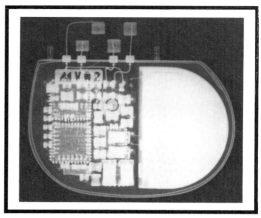

1. **IDENTIFICATION/INFORMATION**

Model:	Symbios, Model 7008
24-Hr Telephone Number:	1-800-328-2518
Method of Operation (ICHD code):	DDD, CN/B
Cost:	$6000 (1985)

2. **SPECIAL FEATURES:** DDD bradycardia pacing, with atrial burst (overdrive) and dual demand (underdrive) modalities to suppress detected tachycardias, telemetry, marker channel, electrograms, bipolar, automatic atrial refractory extension, and a tachycardia report.

3. **PROGRAMMABLE FEATURES**

Rate:	40 to 130 ppm (in steps of 10 ppm) for the lower rate; upper rate is programmable from 100 to 175 ppm (in steps of 25 ppm) and the upper rate also functions as the tachycardia rate detection criterion; 135 to 400 ppm (temporary, in steps of 10/20 ppm)
Amplitude (voltage):	2.5 or 5.0 V
Pulse Duration (width):	0.05, .1 to 1.5 msec (steps of .1 msec)
Sensitivity:	0.6, 1.25, 2.5 mV and asynchronous (atrial); 1.25, 2.5, 5.0 mV and asynchronous (ventricular)
Refractory:	155, 225, 325, 400 msec (atrial); 225 (ventricular)—automatic extension to 400 msec and 345 msec, respectively, after a PVC (DDD mode only)
Hysteresis:	none
AV Delay:	25 to 250 msec (steps of 25 msec)
Changes of Mode:	DDD, DDD + Atrial Burst, DDD + A-V Dual Demand, DVI, DVI + Atrial Burst, DVI + A-V Dual Demand, VVI, VVI + Dual Demand, AOO, DOO, VOO
Telemetry Response:	pacemaker ID, status of programmable parameters, battery status, marker channel, and EGM
Other:	programmable ventricular safety pacing, automatic A-V block operation to control propagation of SVTs, temporary programming, temporary burst. Tachycardia modalities require five consecutive P–P or R–R intervals shorter than the programmed upper rate interval before programmed tachycardia therapy begins

4. **ELECTRICAL CHARACTERISTICS**

Sensitivity:	atrial: at a 10-msec sine^2 waveform; and ventricular: at a 40-msec sine^2 waveform

Pulse Duration (width):	from .05 to .2 msec, tolerance is ± 30%; from .3 to 1.5 msec, it is ± 7%
Pulse Amplitude (V):	minimums are 2.1 (half) and 4.6 (full)
Energy (μjoules):	depends on programmed settings
Current Consumption—Basic Rate (ppm):	programmable
Magnet Rate (ppm):	85 (DDD)
Pulse Interval Stability:	± 2 ppm
Refractory Period Pacing (msec):	atrial: programmable to 155, 225, 325, 400 (+ 10 and − 20 msec); ventricular: 225 (+ 10 and − 20 msec)
Refractory Period Sensing (msec):	as above, but automatically extends to 400 (atrial) 345 (ventricular) after a PVC
Escape Interval:	same as programmed basic rate
Rate Hysteresis:	none

5. POWER SOURCE

Number of Cells:	1
Manufacturer/Model Number:	Promeon/Beta 263
Major Chemicals:	lithium iodine
Voltage (each cell):	2.8
Capacity:	2.6 amp-hr (available); 2.0 amp-hr (deliverable)

6. LONGEVITY INFORMATION

Warranty:	limited warranty, 4 yr

7. POWER SOURCE DEPLETION INDICATOR

Change in Pulse Rate:	in DDD mode, to 75 ppm at stage 1 and to 65 ppm at stage 2
Change in Pulse Width:	automatic increase to maintain a nearly constant energy per pulse, as amplitude decreases
Other:	reverts to VVI at stage 2; telemetry reports both stages

8. METHOD FOR PERIODIC TEST OF PROPER FUNCTION

Magnet Test Rate:	85 ppm in DDD mode
Other Changes:	threshold margin test, with 3 paired pulses 10% faster than the magnet rate, with the width of the third pulses reduced by 25%
Recommended Test Frequency:	physician option
Orientation of Magnet or Programmer When Applied to Pacer:	against skin, over and parallel to the generator
Does Magnet Work if Pacer Is Upside Down:	yes
Is Special Magnet Required:	yes, though programming head suffices

9. EFFECT OF ELECTRICAL AND MAGNETIC FIELDS: the bipolar configuration virtually eliminates EMI and myopotential sensing

10. PHYSICAL CHARACTERISTICS

Dimensions (mm):	52 (H) × 60 (L) × 10 (T)
Weight (g):	53
Volume (cc):	23
Materials in Contact With Tissue:	titanium, polyurethane, silicone rubber
Special Implant Position/Procedure:	no special position

11. NONINVASIVE IDENTIFICATION

X-ray Code (radiopaque letters):	VD
Other:	first symbol is Medtronic logo; the number after the letter is the engineering series number

12. TERMINAL CONNECTOR COMPATIBILITY

Medtronic Lead:	in-line, coaxial bipolar
Other:	with adapters
Accepts Atrial and Ventricular:	note that the leads must be inserted into the proper ports for dual-chamber pacing to occur

MEDTRONIC, INC.

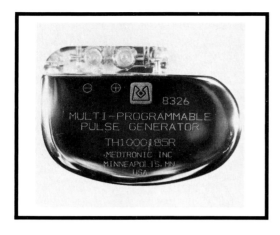 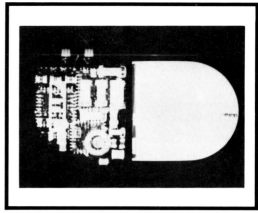

1. **IDENTIFICATION/INFORMATION**

Model:	Pasys, Models 8320, 8322, 8326 (illustrated), 8328, and 8329
24-Hr Telephone Number:	1-800-328-2518
Method of Operation (ICHD code):	VVI, C
Cost:	not available at time of printing

2. **SPECIAL FEATURES:** all models have real-time telemetry: Telemetry of programmed settings; marker channel telemetry; temporary high rate pacing; programmable unipolar/bipolar configuration (except 8329); and automatic capture (Models 8326/28 only)

3. **PROGRAMMABLE FEATURES**

Rate:	30 to 125 ppm in 1-ppm steps (permanent); 130 to 400 ppm in 5/10/20-ppm steps (temporary)
Amplitude (voltage):	0.8, 1.6, 2.5, 3.3, 4.2, 5.0, 6.0, 8.0
Pulse Duration (width):	0.05 to 2.0 msec (0.05-msec steps to .8 and .1-msec steps thereafter)
Sensitivity:	1.25, 2.5, 5.0 mV
Refractory:	220, 325, 400, and 475 msec
Hysteresis:	off, 40, 50, 60 ppm
Changes of Mode:	VVI (AAI), VVT (AAT), VOO (AOO)
Telemetry Response:	real-time: battery voltage and current, pulse amplitude and width, lead impedance and current, and output energy; status of programmable parameters, battery status, and marker channel
Other:	unipolar/bipolar (only bipolar models) and automatic capture (Models 8326/28 only)

4. **ELECTRICAL CHARACTERISTICS**

Sensitivity:	at a 40-msec sine^2 waveform
Pulse Duration (width):	measured at 0.5 V from baseline
Pulse Amplitude (V):	measured at the leading edge
Energy (μjoules):	varies according to programmed settings
Basic Rate (ppm):	programmable
Magnet Rate (ppm):	same as programmed
Pulse Interval Stability:	± 2 ppm
Refractory Period Pacing (msec):	programmable, ± 20
Refractory Period Sensing (msec):	same as pacing refractory
Escape Interval:	same as programmed rate
Rate Hysteresis:	programmable, ± 2 ppm

5. POWER SOURCE

Number of Cells:	1
Manufacturer/Model Number:	Promeon/Alpha 283
Major Chemical:	lithium iodine
Voltage (each cell):	2.78
Capacity:	2.2 amp-hr (available); 1.7 amp-hr (deliverable)

6. LONGEVITY INFORMATION

Warranty:	lifetime limited on components and workmanship; 10 yr on battery (8 yr, full, and remaining prorated)

7. POWER SOURCE DEPLETION INDICATOR

Change in Pulse Rate:	10% rate decrease from programmed value
Change in Pulse Width:	automatic increase to maintain nearly constant energy per pulse, as amplitude decreases
Other:	two stages; real-time telemetry and permanent programming are cancelled at stage 2.

8. METHOD FOR PERIODIC TEST OF PROPER FUNCTION

Magnet Test Rate:	same as programmed
Other Changes:	threshold margin test, with 3 pulses at 100 ppm, with the third pulse width reduced by 25%
Recommended Test Frequency:	physician option
Orientation of Magnet or Programmer When Applied to Pacer:	against skin, over and parallel to the generator
Does Magnet Work if Pacer Is Upside Down:	yes
Is Special Magnet Required:	yes, though programming head suffices

9. EFFECT OF ELECTRICAL AND MAGNETIC FIELDS: units may, depending on the signal intensity, continue to sense or revert to asynchronous operation

10. PHYSICAL CHARACTERISTICS

Dimensions (mm):	42–46 (H) × 59 (L) × 10 (T)
Weight (g):	40
Volume (cc):	21
Materials in Contact With Tissue:	titanium, polyurethane, silicone rubber
Pulse Generator:	elliptical window in external coating
Surface Area:	approximately 2 in^2 (all models)
Material:	titanium
Special Implant Position/Procedure:	uncoated side to face toward skin

11. NONINVASIVE IDENTIFICATION

X-ray Code (radiopaque letters):	8320 (JU); 8322 (LL); 8326 (TH); 8328 (UD); 8329 (VB)
Other:	first symbol is Medtronic logo; the number after the letters is the engineering series number

12. TERMINAL CONNECTOR COMPATIBILITY

Cordis Lead:	yes (Models 8329, 8328, and 8329)
Medtronic Lead:	yes
Other:	adapters may be needed for others
Accepts Atrial and Ventricular:	yes

MEDTRONIC, INC.

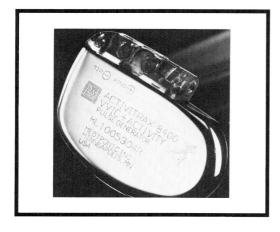
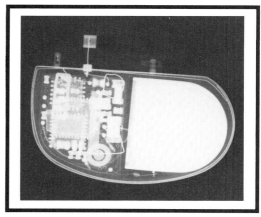

1. **IDENTIFICATION/INFORMATION**

Model:	Activitrax, Models 8400 (illustrated), 8402, and 8403
24-Hr Telephone Number:	1-800-328-2518
Method of Operation (ICHD code):	VVI + Activity, C
Cost:	$4600

2. **SPECIAL FEATURES:** pacing rate changes in response to increase or decrease in patient's activity; telemetry of programmed parameters, battery status, programming confirmation; marker channel; EGM

3. **PROGRAMMABLE FEATURES**

Rate:	40 to 130 ppm (steps of 10 ppm) in VVI; 60, 70, 80 ppm in VVI + Activity
Amplitude (voltage):	2.5 V (half); 5.0 V (full)
Pulse Duration (width):	.05, .1 to 1.5 msec (steps of .1 msec)
Sensitivity:	1.25, 2.5, 5.0 mV and asynchronous
Refractory:	225 msec
Hysteresis:	off, 40 and 50 ppm (VVI mode only)
Changes of Mode:	VVI (AAI) + Activity; VOO (AOO) + Activity; VVI (AAI); VOO (AOO)
Telemetry Response:	pacemaker ID, status of programmable parameters, battery status, programming confirmation, marker channel, EGM
Other:	programmable activity threshold (3 settings—low, medium, and high), programmable rate response (10 settings), and maximum activity rate (100, 125, and 150 ppm)

4. **ELECTRICAL CHARACTERISTICS**

Sensitivity:	at a 40-msec sine^2 waveform; ± 20%
Pulse Duration (width):	± 10%
Pulse Amplitude (V):	± 10%
Energy (μjoules):	depends on programmed settings
Basic Rate (ppm):	programmable, ± 1%
Magnet Rate (ppm):	85 (in VVI + Activity); programmed rate in VVI
Pulse Interval Stability:	± 1%
Refractory Period Pacing (msec):	nonprogrammable (225)
Refractory Period Sensing (msec):	same as pacing refractory
Escape Interval:	same as programmed (VVI) rate
Rate Hysteresis:	programmable ± 1%

5. **POWER SOURCE**

Number of Cells:	1
Manufacturer/Model Number:	Promeon/Alpha 283
Major Chemical:	lithium iodine
Voltage (each cell):	2.78
Capacity:	2.2 amp-hr available, with 1.7 amp-hr deliverable

6. **LONGEVITY INFORMATION**

Warranty:	lifetime limited warranty on components and workmanship; 10 yr on battery (8 yr, full, and remaining prorated)

7. **POWER SOURCE DEPLETION INDICATOR**

Change in Pulse Rate:	65 ppm
Change in Pulse Width:	automatic increase to maintain a nearly constant energy per pulse, as amplitude decreases
Other:	reverts to VVI (without Activity) telemetry reports battery status

8. **METHOD FOR PERIODIC TEST OF PROPER FUNCTION**

Magnet Test Rate:	85 ppm (VVI + Activity); same as programmed rate in VVI (without Activity)
Other Changes:	threshold margin test, with 3 pulses at 100 ppm, with the pulse width of the third pulse reduced by 25%
Recommended Test Frequency:	physician option
Orientation of Magnet or Programmer When Applied to Pacer:	against skin, over and parallel to the pulse generator
Does Magnet Work if Pacer Is Upside Down:	yes
Is Special Magnet Required:	yes, though programming head suffices

9. **EFFECT OF ELECTRICAL AND MAGNETIC FIELDS:** the bipolar units (8400 and 8402) are usually not subject to EMI, whereas the unipolar unit (8403), depending on the signal strength, may continue sensing, revert to asynchronous operation, or pace at an altered rate. Muscle contractions, when detected by the activity sensor, may alter the pacing rate

10. **PHYSICAL CHARACTERISTICS**

Dimensions (mm):	42 and 46 (H) $\times$ 59 (L) $\times$ 10 (T)
Weight (g):	40
Volume (cc):	20
Materials in Contact With Tissue:	titanium, polyurethane, silicone
Pulse Generator:	elliptical window in the external coating (Model 8403)
Surface Area:	Approximately 2 in^2 (Model 8403)
Material:	titanium
Special Implant Position/Procedure:	uncoated side to face toward skin (8403)

11. **NONINVASIVE IDENTIFICATION**

X-ray Code (radiopaque letters):	8400 (IW); 8402 (IJ); 8403 (IV)
Other:	first symbol is the Medtronic logo; the number after the letter is the engineering series number

12. **TERMINAL CONNECTOR COMPATIBILITY**

Cordis Lead:	yes
Medtronic Lead:	yes
Other:	with adapters
Accepts Atrial and Ventricular:	yes

MEDTRONIC, INC.

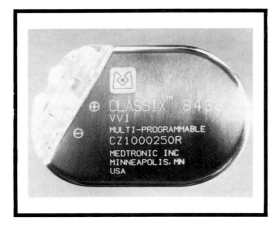 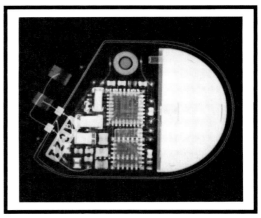

1. IDENTIFICATION/INFORMATION

Model:	Classix, Models 8436, 8437, 8438 (illustrated)
24-Hr Telephone Number:	1-800-328-2518
Method of Operation (ICHD code):	VVI, C
Cost:	$4500 (1985)

2. SPECIAL FEATURES: very small size; anatomical shape; telemetry; battery status; electrogram; 10-second ECG via programmer

3. PROGRAMMABLE FEATURES

Rate:	30 to 129 in 1-ppm steps (permanent); 130 to 400 ppm in 10/20-ppm steps (temporary)
Amplitude (voltage):	2.5 (half); 5.0 (full)
Pulse Duration (width):	0.05, 1.0 to 2.0 msec in 0.1-msec steps
Sensitivity:	1.25, 2.5, 5.0 mV
Refractory:	228, 325, 400 msec
Hysteresis:	off, 40, 50, 60 ppm
Changes of Mode:	VVI (AAI), VVT (AAT), VOO (AOO)
Telemetry Response:	all programmed parameters, battery status, programming confirmation, and EGM

4. ELECTRICAL CHARACTERISTICS

Sensitivity:	programmable
Pulse Duration (width):	programmable
Pulse Amplitude (V):	programmable
Refractory Period Pacing (msec):	programmable
Refractory Period Sensing (msec):	programmable
Escape Interval:	same as programmed rate
Rate Hysteresis:	programmable

5. POWER SOURCE

Number of Cells:	1
Manufacturer/Model Number:	Promeon/Zeta 205
Major Chemicals:	lithium iodine
Capacity:	.9 amp-hr available, .6 amp-hr deliverable

6. LONGEVITY INFORMATION

Warranty:	lifetime limited on components and workmanship; 10 yr on battery (first 5 yr full, with last 5 prorated)

7. POWER SOURCE DEPLETION INDICATOR

Changes in Pulse Rate:	10% rate decrease
Changes in Pulse Width:	automatic increase to maintain a nearly constant energy per pulse, as amplitude decreases

8. METHOD FOR PERIODIC TEST OF PROPER FUNCTION

Magnet Test Rate:	10% rate decrease from programmed
Other Changes:	threshold margin test, with 3 pulses at 100 ppm, with the width of the third pulse reduced by 25%
Recommended Test Frequency:	physician option
Orientation of Magnet or Programmer When Applied to Pacer:	against skin, slightly offset from and parallel to the pacemaker
Does Magnet Work if Pacer Is Upside Down:	it may not
Is Special Magnet Required:	yes, though programming head suffices

9. EFFECT OF ELECTRICAL AND MAGNETIC FIELDS: bipolar models are virtually immune to sensing of EMI and myopotentials; unipolar model, depending on the signal's intensity, may continue sensing or revert to asynchronous operation

10. PHYSICAL CHARACTERISTICS

Dimensions (mm):	41 (H) $\times$ 61–63 (L) $\times$ 6 (T)
Weight (g):	28
Volume (cc):	13
Materials in Contact With Tissue:	titanium, polyurethane, silicone rubber
Pulse Generator:	elliptical window in external coating of Model 8437
Surface Area:	approximately 2 in^2 (Model 8437)
Material:	titanium
Special Implant Position/Procedure:	uncoated side (Model 8437) facing toward skin

11. NONINVASIVE IDENTIFICATION

X-ray Code (radiopaque letters):	8436 (GS); 8437 (CX); 8438 (CZ)
Other:	first symbol is Medtronic logo; the number after the letters is the engineering series number

12. TERMINAL CONNECTOR COMPATIBILITY

Cordis Lead:	yes
Medtronic Lead:	yes
Other:	yes, with adapters
Accepts Atrial and Ventricular:	yes

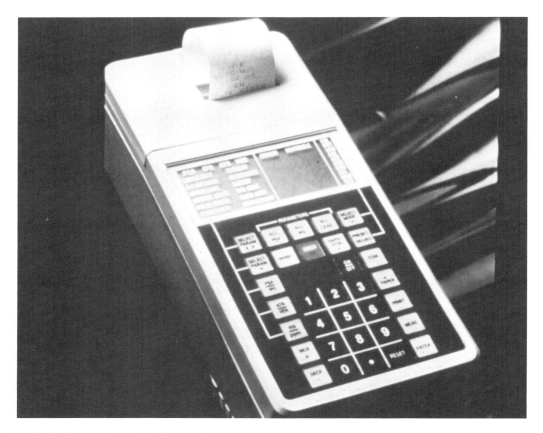

MANUFACTURER: Medtronic, Inc.

MODEL: 5311A-V PSA (pacing system analyzer)

1. **Current Output:**   0 to 25.0 mA

2. **Voltage Output:**   0.1 to 10.0 V

3. **Pulse Duration:**   0.05 to 2.0 msec

4. **Fixed Rate:**   30 to 180 ppm

5. **Sensitivity (pacing):**   0.75 to 10.0 mV (atrial), 1.0 to 10.0 mV (ventricular)

6. **Refractory Period:**   Determined by selecting pacing mode as follows:

Mode	Atrial Refractory Period	Ventricular Refractory Period
VVI		325 msec
VVT		325 msec
AAI	400 msec	
AAT	400 msec	
DDD	235 msec	233 msec
DVI		233 msec
VDD	225 msec	225 msec

7. **Sensing Threshold Sensitivity:**   Directly measures P-wave and R-wave signal amplitudes within the range of 0.5 to 25.4 mV

8. **Output Sample Point:**   Amplitude measured at peak, pulse duration measured at 0.5 volts amplitude

9. **Battery Replacement Indicator:**   "BATTERY LOW" message on display

10. **Power Supply:**   Four 9-V alkaline batteries (Eveready 522 or equivalent)

11. **Battery Life:**   10 hours

12. **Display:**   Multifunction liquid crystal

13. **Size:**   22.9 × 10.1 × 8.6 cm

14. **Weight:**   1.5 kg (3.3 lb)

15. **Special Features:**   Ten selectable pacing modes include dual-chamber options:

VVI	AOO
VVT	DDD (unipolar)
VOO	DVI (unipolar)
AAI	DOO (unipolar)
AAT	VDD (unipolar)

Dual-chamber pacing includes adjustable upper rate and AV interval:

Upper Rate:	100 to 180 ppm
AV Interval:	2.5 to 250 msec

Measurable parameters for lead system analysis:

Output Voltage:	0.5 to 10.2 V
Lead Current:	0.1 to 25 mV
Lead Resistance:	200 to 1999 ohms
Pulse Energy:	1.0 to 1000 μJ
P-Wave Amplitude:	0.5 to 25.4 mV
R-Wave Amplitude:	0.5 to 25.4 mV
P- or R-Wave Signal Slew Rate:	0.1 to 7.5 V/sec

Measurable parameters in pacemaker test mode:

Rate:	30 to 1999 ppm
Rate Interval:	1999 to 30 msec
A-V Interval:	2.5 to 250 msec
Upper Rate:	100 to 180 ppm
Upper Rate Interval:	600 to 333 msec
Output Voltage:	1.0 to 10.2 V (peak)
Pulse Duration:	0.05 to 19.99 msec
Sensitivity:	0.5 to 10.0 mV
Pulse Current:	0.2 to 20.4 mA (peak)*
Pulse Energy:	1.0 to 1000 μJ*
Refractory Period:	50 to 1000 msec

Other special features:
Integral printer with graphics capability provides:
—Hard copy of all set and measured parameter values
—Atrial or ventricular electrogram annotated with signal slew rate and peak-to-peak voltage values
Atrial electrogram has feature to aid testing for retrograde conduction.
Rapid stimulation to 800 ppm
Output inhibit function
Emergency VVI pacing override (a one-keystroke safety feature)

---

* Based on 500 ohm internal load.

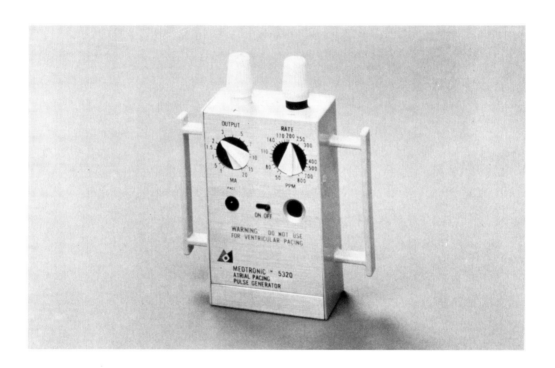

MANUFACTURER: Medtronic, Inc.

MODEL: 5320 External Generator

1. **Rate Range:**   50 to 800 ppm, continuously adjustable

2. **Rate Calibration Accuracy:**   ± 10% of the rate indicated on dial

3. **Output Current Range:**   continuously adjustable from 0.1 to 20 mA; current at any setting is constant regardless of load, to a maximum of 10 volts as measured at output terminals across 500 ohms

4. **Current Calibration Accuracy:**   ± 10% of value indicated on dial (0.5 to 20 mA)

5. **Pulse Width:**   2.0 ± 0.4 msec

6. **Power Source:**   battery; Mallory TR 146X, Eveready E146X, or equivalent

7. **Power Life:**   110 hr at maximum rate and amplitude

8. **Physical Dimensions:**   6.7 cm (2.6 in) × 11.4 cm (4.5 in) × 3.7 cm (1.5 in), excluding handles and terminals

9. **Weight (including battery):**   340 g

10. **Price:** $1400

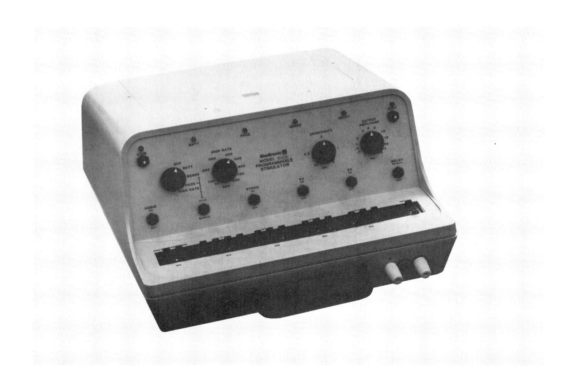

MEDTRONIC, INC.

1. **MODEL:**   5326 Programmable Stimulator for Cardiac Electrophysiologic Studies

2. **TIMING**

High Rate:	50 ppm to 800 ppm $+/-$ 10% of dial setting
S_1–S_1 Interval:	200 msec to 1999 msec $+/-$ 1 msec
S_1–S_2 Interval:	1 msec to 999 msec $+/-$ 1 msec
S_2–S_3 Interval:	1 msec to 999 msec $+/-$ 1 msec
S_3–S_4 Interval:	1 msec to 999 msec $+/-$ 1 msec
Delay:	1 sec to 9 sec $+/-$ 0.1 sec

NOTE: The escape interval following a premature stimulus equals the selected delay time plus the S_1–S_1 interval.

3. **OUTPUT**

Pulse Duration:	0.1 msec to 1.9 msec $\pm$ 0.05 msec (PACE mode or premature stimuli), 1.8 msec $\pm$ 0.2 msec fixed (HIGH RATE mode only)
Pulse Amplitude Range:	0.1 mA to 28 mA (500 ohm load)
Pulse Amplitude Accuracy:	$+/-$ 10% of dial setting or 0.2 mA (whichever is greater) derated 1% degree deviation from 70°F

4. **POWER SOURCE:** 1.5 volt, size C alkaline cells, nine required (NEDA type 14A). Expected battery life is greater than 40 operating hours with nominal pacing parameters: 70 ppm at 10 mA into a 500 ohm load

5. **SENSING**

Calibration Signal:	15-msec sine^2 waveform (isolated 0.5 cycle)
Adjustable Range:	0.2 mV to 20 mV
Accuracy:	$+/-$ 30% of dial indication derated 1%/mV/degree deviation from 70°F
Refractory:	250 msec $+/-$ 75 msec

6. **TEMPERATURE**

Operating:	50°F to 110°F (10°C to 44°C)

7. **DIMENSIONS:**   13.0 in $\times$ 13.5 in $\times$ 7.5 in

8. **WEIGHT:**   approximately 9.5 lb (with batteries)

9. **PRICE:** $8000

10. **APPLICATIONS**

This Model 5326 programmable stimulator has applications in electrophysiologic studies where electrical stimulation of the heart is used for:
- refractory measurements
- initiation of re-entrant tachyarrhythmias
- termination of re-entrant tachyarrhythmias
- sinus node overdrive
- location of accessory pathways
- testing for conduction system disorders

11. **FEATURES**
- Up to 3 premature stimuli
- Digitally adjustable provocative pacing intervals
- Synchronous or asynchronous pacing
- Synchronous or asynchronous burst pacing up to 800 ppm
- Output amplitude adjustable up to 28 mA
- Adjustable delay between pacing protocols
- Battery-powered, portable
- Audiovisual indicators for pace, sense, delay, stimulation, standby, and battery condition
- Programmable paper recorder start/stop trigger

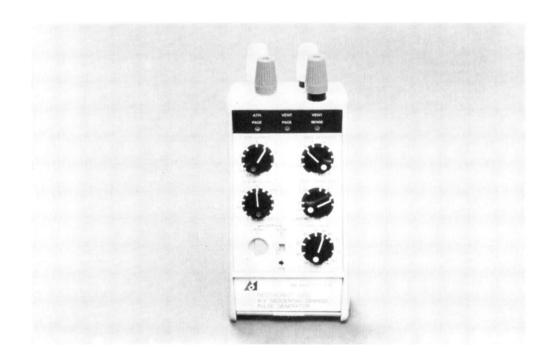

MANUFACTURER: Medtronic, Inc.

MODEL: 5330 Dual-Channel External Generator

1. **Rate Range:**   30 to 180 ppm, continuously adjustable in 1-ppm increments

2. **Rate Calibration Accuracy:**   atrial: 0.1 to 20 mA continuously adjustable, constant current; ventricular: 0.1 to 20 mA continuously adjustable, constant current

3. **Output Current Range:**   atrial: 0.1 to 20 mA, constant current, continuously adjustable; ventricular: 0.1 to 20 mA, constant current, continuously adjustable

4. **Current Calibration Accuracy:**   ± 10% at dial settings from 0.5 mA to 10 mA inclusive with loads of 300 ohms to 1200 ohms; ± 20% for dial settings from 10 mA to 20 mA with loads up to 700 ohms; dial accuracy not calibrated below 0.5 mA. Output voltage may be limited to 14 volts

5. **Pulse Width:**   atrial: 1msec; ventricular: 0.80 msec

6. **Sensitivity Range:**   maximum sensitivity 1.0 mV to asynchronous, continuously adjustable

7. **Refractory Period:**   250 msec maximum (after ventricular pulse output or sensed QRS)

8. **Power Source:**   one 9-V alkaline battery

9. **Battery Life:**   at typical rate and output settings of 72 ppm and 10 mA, projected battery life is 500 hours

10. **Physical Dimensions:**   7.5 cm (3 in) × 4.0 cm (1.6 in) × 14.0 cm (5.6 in), excluding terminals

11. **Weight (including battery):**   550 g

12. **Price:** $2400

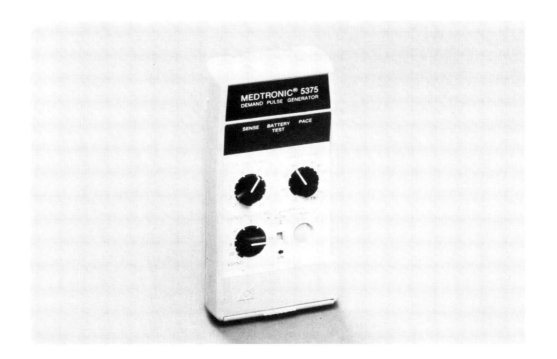

MANUFACTURER: Medtronic, Inc.

MODEL: 5375 Demand Pulse Generator

1. **Rate Range:**   30 to 180 ppm, continuously adjustable in 1-ppm increments

2. **Rate Calibration Accuracy:**   5% of indicated dial rate from 50 to 150 ppm; 10% of indicated dial rate outside these limits

3. **Output Current Range:**   constant current from 0.1 to 20 mA, regardless of load, to a maximum of 18 V

4. **Current Calibration Accuracy:**   ± 10% or 0.25 mA (whichever is greater)* from 0.5 to 20 mA; accuracy not calibrated below 0.5 mA

5. **Pulse Width:**   1.8 + 0.2 msec

6. **Sensitivity Range:**   1.0 mV ± 0.5 mV for a 40-msec, sine-squared pulse

7. **Refractory Period:**   250 msec, initiated by the emission of a pacing pulse or the sensing of an R wave

8. **Power Source:**   9-V alkaline battery, Eveready Energizer 522

9. **Battery Life:**   at 70 ppm and 10 mA, projected battery life using a recommended battery is 500 hours

10. **Physical Dimensions:**   3.8 cm (1.5 in) × 7.6 cm (3 in) × 14.5 cm (5.7 in)

11. **Weight:**   476 g

12. **Price:** $1400

---

* Output current will decrease up to 0.2 mA when the sensitivity dial is rotated from 1 mV to Async.

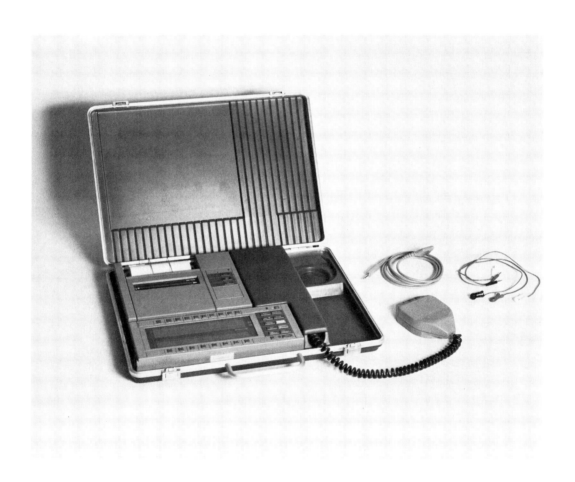

MANUFACTURER: Medtronic, Inc.

MODEL: 9710 Programmer

1. **Carrier Frequency:**   175 kHz

2. **Programming Range:**   0 to 2.0 inches

3. **Display:**   dual displays, multifunction liquid crystal

4. **Programmable Parameters:**

   The programmable parameters, parameter values, and modes and the applicable pacemaker models are determined by a changeable, plug-in software cartridge. New software cartridges keep the Model 9710 programmer current as new pacemaker models and programming functions become available.

   Depending on the pulse generator model, programmable parameters include, but are not limited to, the following:

rate	pulse duration
A-V interval	sensitivity
upper rate	pulse amplitude
hysteresis	refractory period

   Programmable pacing modes include, but are not limited to, the following:

DDD	DVI	DOO	VDD
VVI	VOO	AAI	AOO

   Functions include telemetry of programmed mode and parameter values and battery status. Confirmation of a programming transmission is via telemetry when applicable or by surface signal detection of a program confirmation indicator (coded variation of output pulse timing for one cycle).

5. **Power Source:**   three 9-V alkaline batteries (Eveready 522 or equivalent)

6. **Pacemaker Series:**   all current Medtronic models; see item 4 above

7. **Dimensions:**   5 × 10.9 × 29.2 cm

8. **Weight:**   1.2 lb (0.53 kg) with batteries

9. **Price:** $8000

10. **Special Features:**

    Programmer includes battery-powered printer with graphics capability. The programming system, including the printer, is portable and contained within a 2.5 inch thick, attache-type carrying case.

Programmer is easy to use. Displayed instructions prompt each step of a keystroke sequence.

Special functions include:
- Temporary parameter programming
- ECG printout annotated with Marker Channel telemetry when applicable
- Interrogate function reads pacemaker programmed state and battery status
- Pacemaker output inhibit function
- Direct measurement of output rate, A-V interval, and pulse duration
- Auto threshold measurement function
- One-keystroke programming of nominal or high-output parameters
- Built-in clock and calendar
- Printer functions provide ongoing or summary printouts

PACESETTER SYSTEMS, INC.

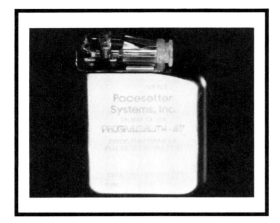
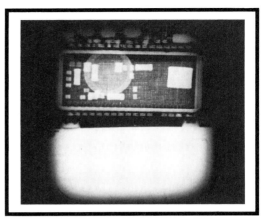

1. **IDENTIFICATION/INFORMATION**

Model:	223 PROGRAMALITH AV
24-Hr Telephone Number:	1-818-362-6822
Method of Operation (ICHD code):	DVI Committed
Cost:	$4395

2. **SPECIAL FEATURES:** 4 asynchronous pacing outputs at the programmed rate post–magnet removal

3. **PROGRAMMABLE FEATURES**

Rate:	45 to 110 ppm
Amplitude (current):	5.0, 2.5, 1.3 V (ventricle only)
Pulse Duration (width):	.2, .4, .8, 1.6 msec
Sensitivity:	1, 2, 4, 8 mV
Refractory:	250, 325, 400, 475 msec
AV Delay:	fixed at 150 msec (105 msec with magnet application)
Changes of Mode (e.g., VVT to VVI):	VOO, VVI, VVT, DVI
Telemetry Response:	both programmed settings and real-time measured data

4. **ELECTRICAL CHARACTERISTICS** (at standard settings)

Sensitivity (mV):	2.0
Pulse Duration (width):	.8 msec
Pulse Amplitude (V):	5.0 V (atrial, fixed), 5.0 V (ventricular)
Energy (μjoules):	33
Current Consumption at 72 ppm 500 ohms (μamps):	23 (VVI), 38 (DVI)
Current Consumption Inhibited (μamps):	6
Basic Rate (ppm):	70
Magnet Rate (ppm):	90 asynchronous (105 msec AV delay) (BOL)
Pulse Interval Stability:	$\pm$ 1 ppm
Refractory Period Pacing (msec):	325
Refractory Period Sensing (msec):	325
Escape Interval:	same as programmed pacing rate
Rate Hysteresis:	none

5. **POWER SOURCE**

Number of Cells:	1
Manufacturer/Model Number:	WGL 761/23
Major Chemicals:	lithium iodine
Voltage (each cell):	2.8
Capacity:	2.5 amp-hr
Total Watt Hours:	7.0

6. LONGEVITY INFORMATION

Warranty:	5 yr replacement agreement
Manufacturer's Projected Life:	9.6 yr (VVI), 5.8 yr (DVI)

7. POWER SOURCE DEPLETION INDICATOR

Change in Pulse Rate:	decrease in magnet rate to 77 ppm
Change in Pulse Width:	25% increase
Other:	telemetered current drain and cell impedance

8. METHOD FOR PERIODIC TEST OF PROPER FUNCTION

Magnet Test Rate:	90 BOL, 77 RRT
Other Changes:	25% increase in pulse width
Recommended Test Frequency:	quarterly
Orientation of Magnet or Programmer When Being Applied to Pacer:	see Figs. A & B (below)
Does Magnet Work if Pacer Is Upside Down:	yes
Is Special Magnet Required:	no

9. EFFECTS OF ELECTRICAL AND MAGNETIC FIELDS: sensed repetitive signals which occur (1) more frequently than 100 msec will result in asynchronous pacing at time programmed rate; (2) less frequently than 100 msec and during the alert period will result in inhibition of the pulse generator output

10. PHYSICAL CHARACTERISTICS

Dimensions (mm):	63 × 47 × 11.7
Weight (g):	68
Volume (cc):	30
Specific Gravity (g/cc):	2.3
Materials in Contact With Tissue:	titanium, epoxy
Surface Area:	750 mm^2
Material:	titanium
Special Implant Position/Procedure:	logo up (indifferent window away from muscle)

11. NONINVASIVE IDENTIFICATION

X-ray Code (radiopaque letters):	none
Other:	horizontal configuration of electronics above battery

12. TERMINAL CONNECTOR COMPATIBILITY

Cordis Lead:	no
Medtronic Lead:	yes
Unipolar:	yes
Bipolar:	no
Accepts Atrial and Ventricular:	yes

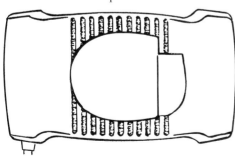

FIGURE A. Programming/telemetry head alignment with respect to pacemaker. NOTE: Do not place programming/telemetry head near a metal surface during programming or interrogation.

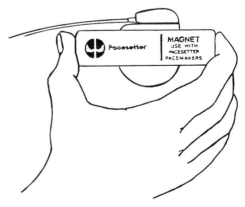

FIGURE B. Test magnet alignment.

PACESETTER SYSTEMS, INC.

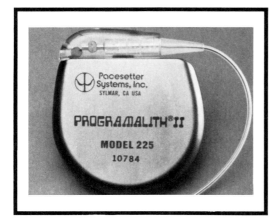
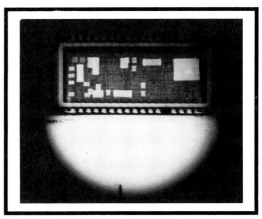

1. IDENTIFICATION/INFORMATION

Model:	225/226 PROGRAMALITH II
24-Hr Telephone Number:	1-818-362-6822
Method of Operation (ICHD code):	SSIM
Cost:	$4195

2. SPECIAL FEATURES: 4 asynchronous pacing outputs at the programmed rate post–magnet removal

3. PROGRAMMABLE FEATURES

Rate:	45 to 110 ppm
Amplitude (current):	1.3, 2.5, 5.0 V
Pulse Duration (width):	.2, .4, .8, 1.6 msec
Sensitivity:	1.0, 2.0, 4.0, 8.0 mV
Refractory:	250, 325, 400, 475 msec
Hysteresis:	0, 120, 300, 600 msec
Telemetry Response:	programmed settings and real-time measured data

4. ELECTRICAL CHARACTERISTICS (at standard settings)

Sensitivity (mV):	2.0
Pulse Duration (width):	.8 msec
Pulse Amplitude (V):	5.0
Energy (μjoules):	33
Current Consumption at 72 ppm 500 ohms (μamps):	23
Current Consumption Inhibited (μamps):	6
Basic Rate (ppm):	70
Magnet Rate (ppm):	5% below programmed rate (BOL)
Pulse Interval Stability:	± 1 ppm
Refractory Period Pacing (msec):	325
Refractory Period Sensing (msec):	325
Escape Interval:	same as programmed pacing rate
Rate Hysteresis:	0 msec

5. POWER SOURCE

Number of Cells:	1
Manufacturer/Model Number:	WGL 8077
Major Chemicals:	lithium iodine
Voltage (each cell):	2.8
Capacity:	1.8 amp-hr
Total Watt Hours:	5.0 WH

6. LONGEVITY INFORMATION

Warranty:	lifetime replacement agreement
Manufacturer's Projected Life:	9.6 yr

7. POWER SOURCE DEPLETION INDICATOR

Change in Pulse Rate:	decrease in magnet rate to 10% below programmed rate
Change in Pulse Width:	25% increase
Other:	telemetered current drain and cell impedance

8. METHOD FOR PERIODIC TEST OF PROPER FUNCTION

Magnetic Test Rate:	5% below programmed rate at BOL and 10% below programmed rate at RRT
Recommended Test Frequency:	quarterly
Orientation of Magnet or Programmer When Being Applied to Pacer:	see Figs. A & B
Does Magnet Work if Pacer Is Upside Down:	yes
Is Special Magnet Required:	no

9. EFFECTS OF ELECTRICAL AND MAGNETIC FIELDS: sensed repetitive signals which occurs: (1) more frequently than 150 msec will result in asynchronous pacing at the programmed rate, (2) less frequently than 250 msec but more frequently than the programmed rate will result in inhibition of the pulse generator output

10. PHYSICAL CHARACTERISTICS

Dimensions (mm):	58 × 51 × 11 (225); 61 × 51 × 11 (226)
Weight (g):	60 (225); 63 (226)
Volume (cc):	23 (225); 25 (226)
Specific Gravity (g/cc):	2.5
Materials in Contact With Tissues:	titanium, epoxy

11. NONINVASIVE IDENTIFICATION

X-ray Code (radiopaque letters):	none
Other:	horizontal configuration of electronics above battery

12. TERMINAL CONNECTOR COMPATIBILITY

Cordis Lead:	225 (all 6-mm connectors)
Medtronic Lead:	226 (all 6-mm connectors)
Unipolar:	225
Bipolar:	226
Accepts Atrial and Ventricular:	no

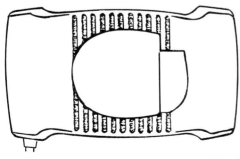

FIGURE A. Programming/telemetry head alignment with respect to pacemaker. NOTE: Do not place programming/telemetry head near a metal surface during programming or interrogation.

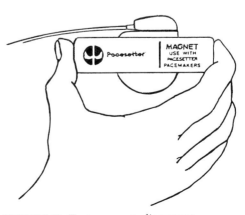

FIGURE B. Test magnet alignment.

PACESETTER SYSTEMS, INC.

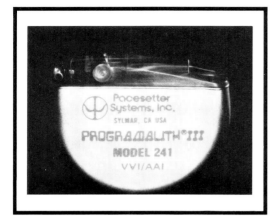 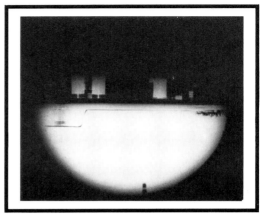

1. IDENTIFICATION/INFORMATION

Model:	241/242 Programalith III
24-Hr Telephone Number:	1-818-362-6822
Method of Operation (ICHD code):	SSIM
Cost:	$4495

2. SPECIAL FEATURES

3. PROGRAMMABLE FEATURES

Rate:	temporary 30, 45, 50, 55, 60, 65, 70, 75, 80, 85, 92, 100, 110 ppm
Amplitude (current):	1.3, 2.5, 5.0, 7.5 V
Pulse Duration (width):	.2, .4, .8, 1.6 msec
Sensitivity:	1.0, 2.0, 4.0, 8.0 mV
Refractory:	250, 325, 400, 475 msec
Hysteresis:	0, 120, 300, 600 msec
Telemetry Response:	programmed settings and real-time measured data

4. ELECTRICAL CHARACTERISTICS (at standard settings)

Sensitivity (mV):	2.0
Pulse Duration (width):	.8
Pulse Amplitude (V):	5.0
Energy (μjoules):	33
Current Consumption at 72 ppm 500 ohms (μamps):	23
Current Consumption Inhibited (μamps):	6
Basic Rate (ppm):	70
Magnet Rate (ppm):	same as programmed rate
Pulse Interval Stability:	± 1%
Refractory Period Pacing (msec):	325
Refractory Period Sensing (msec):	325
Escape Interval:	same as programmed pacing rate
Rate Hysteresis:	0

5. POWER SOURCE

Number of Cells:	1
Manufacturer/Model Number:	WGL 8077
Major Chemicals:	lithium iodine
Voltage (each cell):	2.8
Capacity:	1.8 amp-hr
Total Watt Hours:	5.0

6. LONGEVITY INFORMATION

Warranty:	replacement credit agreement 10-yr full credit period—1%/mo prorata period
Manufacturer's Projected Life:	8 yr (at 100% pacing and STD settings)

7. POWER SOURCE DEPLETION INDICATOR

Change in Pulse Rate:	100-msec increase in pulse interval
Other:	telemetered current drain and cell impedance

8. METHOD FOR PERIODIC TEST OF PROPER FUNCTION

Magnet Test Rate:	same as programmed
Recommended Test Frequency:	quarterly
Does Magnet Work if Pacer Is Upside Down:	yes
Is Special Magnet Required:	no

9. EFFECTS OF ELECTRICAL AND MAGNETIC FIELDS: sensed repetitive signals which occur: (1) more frequently than 100 msec will result in asynchronous pacing at time programmed rate; (2) less frequently than 100 msec and during the alert period will result in inhibition of the pulse generator output

10. PHYSICAL CHARACTERISTICS

Dimensions (mm):	$41 \times 48 \times 8$ (241); $47 \times 48 \times 8$ (242)
Weight (g):	35 (241); 37 (242)
Volume (cc):	15 (241); 16 (242)
Specific Gravity (g/cc):	2.3
Materials in Contact With Tissue:	titanium, epoxy, silicone
Surface Area:	750 mm^2
Material:	titanium
Special Implant Position/Procedure:	logo up (indifferent window away from muscle)

11. NONINVASIVE IDENTIFICATION

X-ray Code (radiopaque letters):	no
Other:	half-moon battery configuration

12. TERMINAL CONNECTOR COMPATIBILITY

Cordis Lead:	no
Medtronic Lead:	yes (all 5-mm connectors)
Unipolar:	241
Bipolar:	242
Accepts Atrial and Ventricular:	no

PACESETTER SYSTEMS, INC.

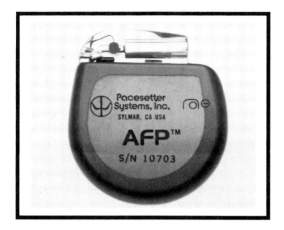 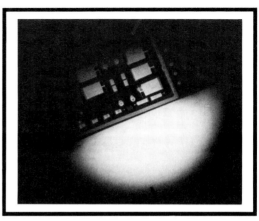

1. IDENTIFICATION/INFORMATION

Model:	261/262
24-Hr Telephone Number:	1-818-362-6822
Method of Operation (ICHD code):	SSIM
Cost:	$4595

2. SPECIAL FEATURES: four asynchronous pacing outputs at the programmed rate post–magnet removal

3. PROGRAMMABLE FEATURES

Rate:	45 to 108 (1-ppm steps); 108 to 118 (2-ppm steps); temporary rate 30
Amplitude (current):	.75, .90, 1.0, 1.3, 1.5, 1.8, 2.0, 2.5, 3.0, 3.5, 4.0, 5.0, 6.0, 7.0, 8.5, 10.0 V
Pulse Duration (width):	.1 to 1.6 msec (.1-msec steps)
Sensitivity:	.5, .6, .8, 1.0, 1.2, 1.5, 2.0, 2.5, 3.0, 4.0, 5.0, 6.0, 7.0, 9.0, 11.0, 14.0 mV
Refractory:	250, 325, 400, 475 msec
Hysteresis:	1 to 40 ppm (1-ppm steps)
Changes of Mode (e.g., VVT to VVI):	AAI/VVI, AAT/VVT, AOO/VOO, off
Telemetry Response:	memory data, real-time measured data, programmed data

4. ELECTRICAL CHARACTERISTICS (at standard settings)

Sensitivity (mV):	2.0
Pulse Duration (width):	0.6
Pulse Amplitude (V):	5.0
Energy (μjoules):	25
Current Consumption at 72 ppm 500 ohms (μamps):	19
Current Consumption Inhibited (μamps):	6
Basic Rate (ppm):	70
Magnet Rate (ppm):	programmable response—on/off 14% higher than programmed prior to RRT. 11% lower than programmed at RRT
Pulse Interval Stability:	±1%
Refractory Period Pacing (msec):	325
Refractory Period Sensing (msec):	325
Escape Interval:	same as programmed pacing rate
Rate Hysteresis:	0

5. POWER SOURCE

Number of Cells:	1
Manufacturer/Model Number:	WGL 8074
Major Chemicals:	lithium iodine
Voltage (each cell):	2.8
Capacity:	2.3 amp-hr
Total Watt Hours:	6.44

6. LONGEVITY INFORMATION

Warranty:	10-yr limited warranty
Manufacturer's Projected Life:	10 yr

7. POWER SOURCE DEPLETION INDICATOR

Change in Pulse Rate:	decrease in magnetic rate to 11% below programmed rate.
Change in Pulse Width:	none
Change in Pulse Amplitude:	none
Other:	telemetered cell voltage

8. METHOD FOR PERIODIC TEST OF PROPER FUNCTION

Magnet Test Rate:	14% higher than programmed prior to RRT. 11% lower than programmed at RRT.
Recommended Test Frequency:	quarterly
Orientation of Magnet or Programmer When Being Applied to Pacer:	see Figs. A & B attached
Does Magnet Work if Pacer Is Upside Down:	yes
Is Special Magnet Required:	no

9. EFFECTS OF ELECTRICAL AND MAGNETIC FIELDS: sensed repetitive signals: (1) above 10 Hz will result in asynchronous pacing at the programmed rate; (2) below 10 Hz and within alert period will result in inhibition of the pulse generator output

10. PHYSICAL CHARACTERISTICS

Dimensions (mm):	54 × 48 × 10.5 (261); 58 × 48 × 10.5 (262)
Weight (g):	50
Volume (cc):	22
Specific Gravity (g/cc):	2.3
Materials in Contact With Tissue:	titanium, hysol epoxy, silicone rubber
Surface Area:	1000 mm^2 (261)
Material:	titanium
Special Implant Position/Procedure:	logo up (window away from muscle)

11. NONINVASIVE IDENTIFICATION

X-ray Code (radiopaque letters):	none
Others:	semicircular battery configuration

12. TERMINAL CONNECTOR COMPATIBILITY

Cordis Lead:	261 (6-mm connector)
Medtronic Lead:	262 (5-mm connector)
Unipolar:	261
Bipolar:	262
Both:	no
Accepts Atrial and Ventricular:	no

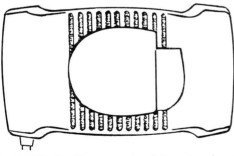

FIGURE A. Programming/telemetry head alignment with respect to pacemaker. NOTE: Do not place programming/telemetry head near a metal surface during programming or interrogation.

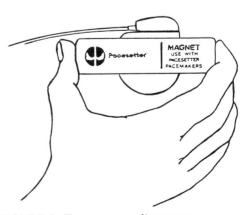

FIGURE B. Test magnet alignment.

PACESETTER SYSTEMS, INC.

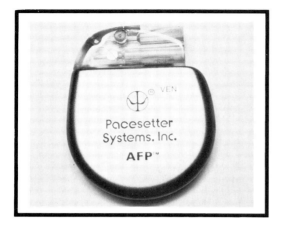
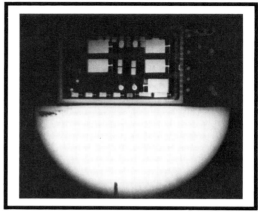

1. IDENTIFICATION/INFORMATION

Model:	AFP Series 273/275/281/283
24-Hr Telephone Number:	1-818-362-6822
Method of Operation (ICHD code):	DVI-DDI/VDD/DDD/DDD
Cost:	$4695/$4595/$5495/$5595

2. SPECIAL FEATURES: four asynchronous pacing outputs at the programmed rate post–magnet removal

3. PROGRAMMABLE FEATURES

Rate:	temporary 30 ppm, 45 to 108 ppm (1-ppm steps), 108 to 118 ppm (2-ppm steps)
Amplitude (current):	.75, .9, 1.3, 1.5, 1.8, 2.0, 2.5, 3.0, 3.5, 4.0, 5.0, 6.0, 7.0, 8.5, 10 V
Pulse Duration (width):	.1 to 1.6 msec (.1-msec steps)
Sensitivity:	.5, .6, .8, 1.0, 1.2, 1.5, 2.0, 2.5, 3.0, 4.0, 5.0, 6.0, 7.0, 9.0, 11, 14 mV
Refractory:	(V) 150, 250, 325, 400, 475; (A) 150, 250, 325, 400, 475, 500
Hysteresis:	equal to or less than the programmed basic rate (1-ppm steps), maximum difference of 40 ppm
AV Delay:	65, 90, 115, 140, 165, 190, 215, 240 msec
Changes of Mode (e.g., VVT to VVI):	*Model 273:* VOO, AOO, VVI, AAI, off, VVT, AAT, DOO, DVI, DDI; *Model 275:* VOO, VVI, VVT, VDD, off; *Model 281:* AAI, AAT, AOO, DDD, VVI, VOO, VDD, DVI, DOO, off; *Model 283:* AAI, AAT, AOO, DDD, VVI, VVT, VOO, VDD, DVI, DDX, DOO, off
Telemetry Response:	identification, programmed settings and real-time measured data
Other:	magnetic response programmable (on/off)

4. ELECTRICAL CHARACTERISTICS (at standard settings)

Sensitivity (mV):	(V) 2 mV, (A) 1 mV
Pulse Duration (width):	.6 msec
Pulse Amplitude (V):	5.0
Energy (μ joules):	25
Current Consumption at 72 ppm 500 ohms (μamps):	32
Current Consumption Inhibited (μamps):	6
Basic Rate (ppm):	70
Magnet Rate (ppm):	14% above programmed basic rate prior to RRT; 11% below programmed basic rate at RRT (when programmed "on")

Pulse Interval Stability:	$\pm$ 1%
Refractory Period Pacing (msec):	(V) 250, (A) 150
Refractory Period Sensing (msec):	(V) 250, (A) 150
Escape Interval:	same as programmed pacing rate
Rate Hysteresis:	0 msec

5. POWER SOURCE

Number of Cells:	1
Manufacturer/Model Number:	Wilson Greatbatch, Ltd, 8074
Major Chemicals:	lithium iodine
Voltage (each cell):	2.8
Capacity:	2.3 amp-hr
Total Watt Hours:	6.4

6. LONGEVITY INFORMATION

Warranty:	*Models 273 & 275:* limited warranty 10 yr (replacement); *Model 281:* clinical device; *Model 283:* replacement credit agreement—4 yr full credit period + $500 unreimbursed medical—prorated at −2% per month
Manufacturer's Projected Life:	> 7 yr

7. POWER SOURCE DEPLETION INDICATOR

Change in Pulse Rate:	decrease in magnetic rate to 11% below programmed rate
Change in Pulse Width:	none
Change in Pulse Amplitude:	none
Other:	telemetered cell voltage

8. METHOD FOR PERIODIC TEST OF PROPER FUNCTION

Magnet Test Rate:	14% above programmed rate (prior to RRT); 11% below programmed rate (RRT)
Recommended Test Frequency:	quarterly
Orientation of Magnet or Programmer When Being Applied to Pacer:	see Figs. A & B on page S-125
Does Magnet Work if Pacer Is Upside Down:	yes
Is Special Magnet Required:	no

9. EFFECTS OF ELECTRICAL AND MAGNETIC FIELDS: sensed repetitive signals: (1) above 10 Hz will result in asynchronous pacing at the programmed rate; (2) below 10 Hz will result in inhibition of the pulse generator output

10. PHYSICAL CHARACTERISTICS

Dimensions (mm):	58.4 × 48.2 × 10.5
Weight (g):	50
Volume (cc):	22
Specific Gravity (g/cc):	2.3
Materials in Contact With Tissue:	titanium, epoxy, silicone rubber
Surface Area:	1000 mm^2
Material:	titanium
Special Implant Position/Procedure:	logo up (indifferent window away from muscle)

11. NONINVASIVE IDENTIFICATION

X-ray Code (radiopaque letters):	no
Others:	half-circle battery configuration

12. TERMINAL CONNECTOR COMPATIBILITY

Cordis Lead:	no
Medtronic Lead:	yes (5-mm connectors)
Unipolar:	yes
Bipolar:	no
Both:	no
Accepts Atrial and Ventricular:	yes

SIEMENS-ELEMA

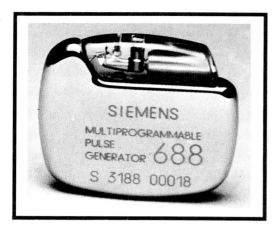 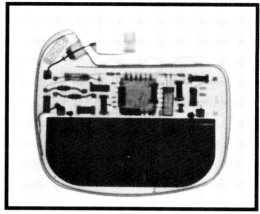

1. IDENTIFICATION/INFORMATION

Model:	688
24-Hr Telephone Number:	1-322-397-5950, 1-800-323-0619
Method of Operation (ICHD code):	VVI, AAI, VOO, AOO
Cost:	$3495 (1984)

2. SPECIAL FEATURES: Vario noninvasive threshold test, high output

3. PROGRAMMABLE FEATURES

Rate:	30 to 150 ppm in steps of 5
Amplitude:	2.5, 5, or 10 V
Pulse Duration (width):	0.25, 0.50, 0.75, 1.0 msec
Sensitivity:	1.1, 1.6, 2.1, 2.7, mV
Refractory:	250, 312, 437 msec or infinite
Hysteresis:	0, 125, 250, 375 msec

4. ELECTRICAL CHARACTERISTICS

Sensitivity (mV):	1.1, 1.6, 2.1, 2.7
Pulse Duration (width):	0.25, 0.50, 0.75, 1.0 msec
Pulse Amplitude (V):	2.5, 5, 10
Energy Watts:	at standard 0.75-msec pulse duration and 5-V output = 25 μjoules
Current Consumption at 72 ppm 500 (μamps):	20
Current Consumption Inhibited (μamps):	4
Basic Rate (ppm):	30 to 50 in steps of 5
Magnet Rate (ppm):	100 BOL
Refractory Period Pacing:	250, 312, 437, or infinite
Refractory Period Sensing:	250, 312, 437, or infinite
Escape Interval:	30 to 150 ppm in steps of 5 ppm
Rate Hysteresis:	0, 125, 250, 375 msec

5. POWER SOURCE

Number of Cells:	1
Manufacturer/Model Number:	CRC or WG
Major Chemicals:	lithium iodine
Voltage:	2.8
Capacity:	1.9k amp-hr
Total Watt Hours:	5.32

6. LONGEVITY INFORMATION

Warranty:	lifetime
Manufacturer's Projected Life:	11 yr at nominal setting

7. POWER SOURCE DEPLETION INDICATOR

Change in Pulse Rate: basic rate unaffected throughout recommended service life. 20% drop at basic rate a few months after ERT

Change in Pulse Width: increases to 1.5 msec a few months after ERT

8. METHOD FOR PERIODIC TEST OF PROPER FUNCTION

Magnet Test Rate: 100 ppm for new generator, drops to <85 ppm at ERT

Other Changes: pulse width increases to 1.5 msec a few mo after ERT

Recommended Test Frequency: at physician's discretion

Does Magnet Work if Pacer Is Upside Down: yes

Is Special Magnet Required: no

9. PHYSICAL CHARACTERISTICS

Dimensions (mm): 9.7 × 48 × 53

Weight (g): 39

Volume (cc): 20

Material in Contact With Tissue: epoxy, titanium, and parylene

Material: titanium

Special Implant Position/Procedure: facing the skin

10. NONINVASIVE IDENTIFICATION

X-ray Code (radiopaque letters): S = Siemens-Elema; 2 = year of manufacture; 88 = model designation (688)

11. TERMINAL CONNECTOR COMPATIBILITY

Cordis Lead: unipolar plug-in diameter 6 mm with sleeve adapter. All Cordis-sized terminals available

Accepts Atrial and Ventricular Leads: yes

12. TELEMETRY: no

SIEMENS-ELEMA

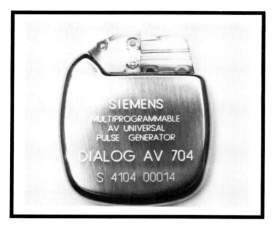 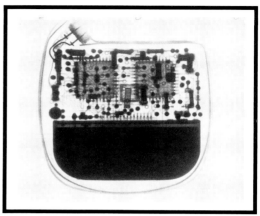

1. IDENTIFICATION/INFORMATION

Model:	Dialog AV 704
24-Hr Telephone Number:	1-312-397-5950, 1-800-323-0619
Method of Operation (ICHD code):	DDD, DVI, VVI, AAI, AOO

2. SPECIAL FEATURES: Vario; noninvasive threshold test in atrium and ventricle

3. PROGRAMMABLE FEATURES

Rate:	30 to 150 in steps of 5 ppm
Amplitude:	A—2.5, 5 V, V—2.5, 5 V
Pulse Duration (width):	0.25, 0.50, 0.75, 1.0 msec, A and V are identical
Sensitivity:	A—0.75, 1.10, 1.5, 1.8 mV; V—1.06, 2.0, 4.0, 8.0 mV
Refractory Period:	A—250, 312, 437; V—250
Hysteresis:	A—0, 125, 250, 375 msec
AV Delay:	10/7, 75/117, 135/180, 200/242
Telemetry Response:	model, serial number, last programming date, program settings, A & V electrograms, event mark paced event counter

4. ELECTRICAL CHARACTERISTICS

Sensitivity (mV):	A—0.75, 1.1, 1.5, 1.8; V—1.0, 2.0, 4.0, 8.0
Pulse Duration (width):	0.25, 0.50, 0.75, 1.0 msec; A & V are identical
Pulse Amplitude (V):	A—2.5, 5; V—2.5, 5
Current Consumption at 72 ppm 500 (µamps):	34 µamps at rate 70, A & V output 5 V pulse 0.5 msec
Current Consumption Inhibited (µamps):	10
Basic Rate (ppm):	30–150 in steps of 5
Magnet Rate (ppm):	100 at BOL
Refractory Period Pacing:	A—250, 312, 437; V—250
Refractory Period Sensing:	A—250, 312, 437; V—250
Escape Interval:	30 to 150 in steps of 5
Rate Hysteresis:	0, 125, 250, 375 msec (atrial hysteresis)

5. POWER SOURCE

Number of Cells:	1
Manufacturer/Model Number:	CRC or WG
Major Chemicals:	lithium iodine
Voltage:	2.8
Capacity:	1.9 amp-hr

6. LONGEVITY INFORMATION

Manufacturer's Projected Life:	5 yr

7. POWER SOURCE DEPLETION INDICATOR

Change in Pulse Rate:	basic rate stable throughout recommended service life; 20% drop a few mo after ERT
Change in Pulse Width:	increase to 1.5 msec a few mo after ERT

8. METHOD FOR PERIODIC TEST OF PROPER FUNCTION

Magnet Test Rate:	100 BOL, <85 ERT
Other Changes:	pulse duration increase to 1.5 mo after ERT
Recommended Test Frequency:	at physician's discretion
Does Magnet Work if Pacer Is Upside Down:	yes
Is Special Magnet Required:	no

9. PHYSICAL CHARACTERISTICS

Dimensions (mm):	13 × 53 × 62
Weight (g):	65
Volume (cc):	27
Material in Contact With Tissue:	epoxy, titanium, and parylene
Material:	titanium
Special Implant Position/Procedure:	text of pulse generator facing the skin

10. NONINVASIVE IDENTIFICATION

X-ray Code (radiopaque letters):	S = Siemens-Elema; 4 = year of manufacture; 04 = Model designation

11. TERMINAL CONNECTOR COMPATIBILITY

Cordis Lead:	plugs in directly
Medtronic Lead:	plugs in with adapter sleeve (included)
Unipolar:	2 unipolar plug-in socket 6 mm

12. TELEMETRY: yes

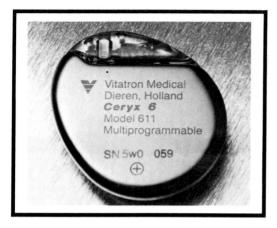
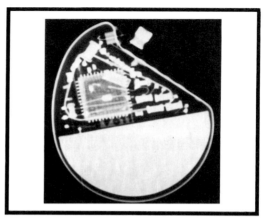
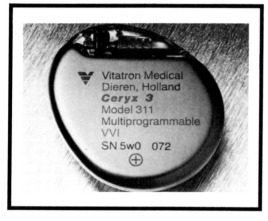
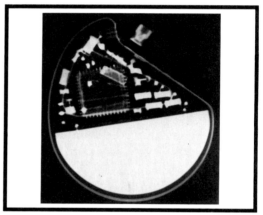

1. IDENTIFICATION/INFORMATION

Model:	Ceryx 6, Model 611; Ceryx 3, Model 311 (illustration only)
24-Hr Telephone Number:	1-800-251-8474
Method of Operation (ICHD code):	SSI, M unipolar

2. SPECIAL FEATURES: voltage step-down mode for threshold measurement, marker channel

3. PROGRAMMABLE FEATURES

Rate:	50, 55, 60, 65, 70 . . . 125 ppm
Amplitude:	2.5, 5.0, 7.5, & 10 Volts
Pulse Duration (width):	0.25, 0.50, 0.75, or 1.0 msec
Sensitivity:	1, 2, 3 or 4 mV
Refractory Period:	37.5, 50, or 62.5% of pacing interval
Hysteresis:	0, 12.5, 25 or 37.5% of pacing interval
Changes of Mode (e.g., VVT to VVI):	VVI, VVT, VOO, AAI, AAT, AOO
Telemetry Response:	see 13 below

4. ELECTRICAL CHARACTERISTICS

Sensitivity (mV):	1, 2, 3, or 4
Pulse Duration (width):	0.25, 0.50, 0.75, or 1.0 msec
Pulse Amplitude (V):	2.5, 5.0, 7.5, 10 Volts
Energy Watts:	50 ± 3 μW
Current Consumption at 70 ppm 500 Ω:	18 ± 1 μA/50 ± 3 μW
Current Consumption Inhibited:	6 ± 1 μA/17 ± 3 μW
Basic Rate (ppm):	50, 55, 60, 65, 70 . . . 125 ppm
Magnet Rate (ppm):	100

Refractory Period:	37.5, 50, or 62.5% of pacing
High Rate Limit:	180 ± 5 ppm

5. POWER SOURCE

Number of Cells:	1
Manufacturer/Model Number:	WGL 8074
Major Chemicals:	LiI_2
Voltage:	2.8
Capacity:	2.3 amp-hr
Total Watt Hours:	6.4

6. LONGEVITY INFORMATION

Manufacturer's Projected Life:	10 yr

7. POWER SOURCE DEPLETION INDICATOR

Change in Pulse Rate:	interval increase: 100 msec
Change in Pulse Amplitude:	5.5 V—5.2 ± 0.1
Other:	magnet interval increase at RRT: 100 msec (magnet rate at RRT: 86)* and telemetry alert to programmer

8. METHOD FOR PERIODIC TEST OF PROPER FUNCTION

Magnet Test Rate:	100 ppm

9. EFFECT OF ELECTRICAL AND MAGNETIC FIELDS: interference rate = programmed rate

10. PHYSICAL CHARACTERISTICS

Dimensions (mm):	57 × 48 × 11
Weight (g):	46
Volume (cc):	24.8
Specific Gravity (g/cc):	1.86
Material in Contact With Tissue:	titanium, epoxy, and silicone rubber

11. NONINVASIVE IDENTIFICATION

X-ray Code (radiopaque letters):	V 611
Other:	D-shaped battery

12. TERMINAL CONNECTOR COMPATIBILITY: accepts all standard 5- to 6-mm connectors

13. TELEMETRY: all pacing parameters, patient code, implantation date, battery status, pacemaker type

14. COMMENT: Specifications for Ceryx 3 Model 311 are the same as described above, except that pulse duration (0.5 msec), refractory period (37.5% of pacing interval), and hysteresis (0) are *not* programmable.

---

*RRT: recommended replacement time

CHAPTER 3

LEADS AND ELECTRODES

Victor Parsonnet, M.D., Alan D. Bernstein, Eng.Sc.D., and Ralph Gallagher

The first cardiac pacemakers were developed independently by several manufacturers. In the United States, Medtronic, Cordis, and Electrodyne were among the earliest pioneers. Naturally, each company had its own system for connecting the pulse generator to the heart, and its own ideas on the type of myocardial electrode that should be used. There was no uniformity in the design and materials used in fabricating the conducting wire, its insulation, the means of connecting it to the pulse generator, or the characteristics of its electrode. In fact, the first pacemaker had no connectors, the lead wire simply being an integral part of the pacemaker—a combined pulse generator, lead, and electrode package. When it became apparent that frequent pacemaker replacement would be necessary, premature battery failure being quite common at the time, the manufacturers sought ways of exchanging the pulse generator without replacing the leads and electrodes. At first, this was accomplished by splicing techniques; later, the obvious idea of a connector of some sort evolved.

Many connector designs were considered, including those shown in Figure 3-1. Because of the neatness and simplicity of the pin-setscrew-and-socket concept, most companies settled on that design, although to this day there is still some variety, particularly in those models developed in Europe.

The general acceptance of the pin-and-socket design soon led to yet another difficulty concerning the use of one manufacturer's lead with another's pulse generator. Not only were the connector sizes incompatible, but the leads and sockets were made of dissimilar metals: if connected together they would induce electrical potentials that would corrode and destroy the connection. Thus, in those days, the wedding of components not designed for each other was discouraged, but not loudly enough for everyone to be aware of the potential danger. Editorials in the medical literature and commentaries in reviews of pacing practice cried out for commonality of connector materials and design. Eventually, the newly formed American Association for Medical Instrumentation (AAMI) directed its Pacemaker Committee to tackle the problem and to formulate standards for pacemaker and lead design. Despite the obvious desirability of its goals, to this day nothing has been accomplished, largely because of the proprietary interests of the manufacturers. Nonetheless, without formal agreements, all pulse generators made in the United States at the time of this writing are equipped with pin-and-socket connectors whose specifications are given in physicians' manuals, and splicers and adapters are available to permit one manufacturer's lead to be connected to another's pulse generator.

Each component of the lead/electrode system has undergone its own evolution. Lead wires began as single-strand conductors, and later were made of several or many strands

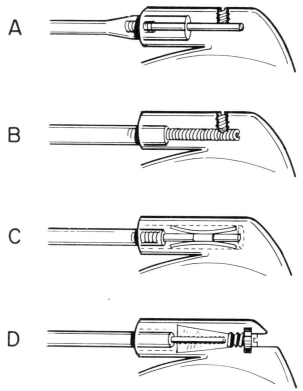

FIGURE 3-1. Diagram of various types of connectors: *(A)* pin in socket; *(B)* bare wire and socket; *(C)* autoclamp; *(D)* chuck.

of steel wire, or of ribbons braided or wound together. These designs finally gave way to the helical-coil configuration (Fig. 3-2) whose central lumen permits the utilization of stiffening wires (stylets) for pervenous implantation techniques. With few exceptions, the multistranded (multifilar) helical coil is the configuration of today's lead, used for both myocardial (epicardial) and pervenous designs.

Lead breakage was common, disturbing, and even dangerous, because of its suddenness and its potentially fatal outcome in patients with fixed complete sinoatrial (SA) block and Stokes-Adams seizures. Thus, there was a vigorous quest for unbreakable leads. Leadless pacemakers were designed but were never used clinically because of the almost insurmountable problem of efficient energy transmission across a spatial barrier. Consideration was given even to implanting an entire nuclear-powered pacemaker within the cavity of the right ventricle, simply to avoid the apparent inevitability of lead fracture.

The multistranded helical steel-alloy conductor became the standard of the day, but even here there was nonuniformity of performance because all steel alloys are not alike. Elgiloy, for example, has less satisfactory long-term survival characteristics than does the DBS (drawn-brazed-stranded) material used by Medtronic and others.

The conductor must be insulated, both for protection from its extremely hostile environment and for electrical isolation of the electrode. Initially, silicone rubber (Silastic) was chosen because of its admirable properties of chemical inertness, impermeability to fluids (but not to water vapor), plasticity, and durability. It lacked only toughness

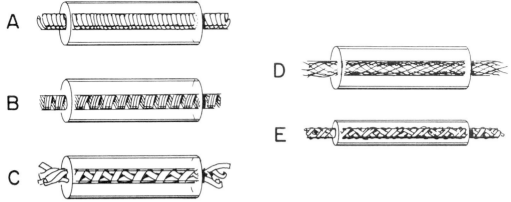

FIGURE 3-2. Diagrammatic representation of five types of conductors: *(A)* helical coil; *(B)* multifilar helical coil; *(C)* ribbons; *(D and E)* fiber-reinforced strands.

and slipperiness, qualities that are desirable to prevent inadvertent damage by the implanter (accidental cutting of insulation during pulse-generator implantation or replacement is not uncommon) and to facilitate the manipulation of one lead alongside another when implanting dual-chamber pacemakers. Later, attention was turned to what was hoped would be the ideal material, polyurethanes of slightly differing chemistries. As has often happened in the history of this field, ideas that seemed good at first did not always prove to be so. In time, at least one of the polyurethanes began to degrade, a process known as environmental stress corrosion. This deterioration has occurred in as many as 18 to 20 percent of the implants, and, when severe enough, it destroys the insulation and the pacing and sensing functions of the lead. The medical (and legal) implications of this problem were extremely serious and remain so today. Nevertheless, some polyurethane-coated leads were excellent, and these have continued to have acceptable if not almost perfect survival records, as shown in Figure 3-3.

Because leads and pulse generators are now readily interchangeable, the user has a wide choice of leads and can select one appropriate to the clinical problems at hand.

The ''business end'' of the lead is its electrode, which should have the following properties:

1. Low stimulation threshold
2. Excellent sensing capability
3. Chemical inertness
4. Resistance to corrosion
5. Means of permanent fixation to the heart
6. Little or no polarization

In hopes of achieving these qualities, a sometimes bewildering variety of electrodes of differing sizes, configurations, and materials has been designed.

It is now conceded that electrodes should be as small as possible (within limits), because the current density at the electrode–tissue interface increases with decreasing electrode size. (The higher the current density, the lower the stimulation threshold and the lower the stimulating current required from the battery.) Electrodes are almost always shaped like spheres, hemispheres, or rings (Figs. 3-4 and 3-5).

Electric current tends to be concentrated at edges and points of an electrode, as it does on a lightning rod, and therefore high current density can be achieved by shaping

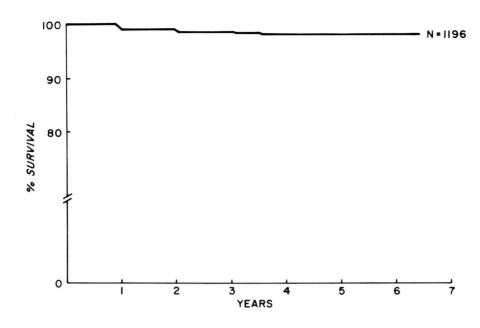

ALL POLYURETHANE LEADS (4/30/85)

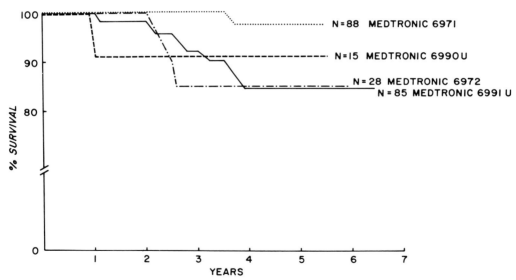

MEDTRONIC POLYURETHANE LEADS (4/30/85)

FIGURE 3-3. *(Top)* Actuarial survival curves of all polyurethane leads used at the Newark Beth Israel Medical Center. *(Bottom)* Actuarial survival curves of specific polyurethane-coated leads. (All leads not shown here have 100 percent actuarial survival.)

the electrode appropriately without making it so sharp that it will perforate the heart. Compromises have become popular, such as layers of concentric rings, like a microscopic pyramid (''target-tipped'' leads), or annuli, disks with open centers. These existing designs meet the requirements listed above and need little further improvement.

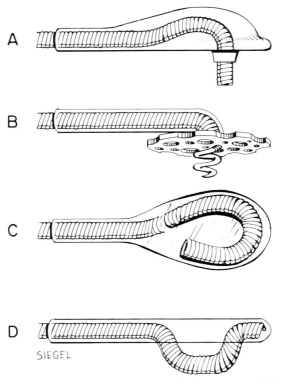

FIGURE 3-4. Epicardial/myocardial electrodes: *(A)* Chardack-type "spike"; *(B)* screw-in electrode with Dacron skirt; *(C and D)* two types of epicardial electrodes, most commonly used for the atrium.

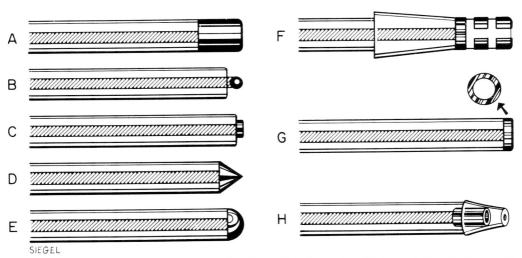

FIGURE 3-5. Diagrams of various types of endocardial electrodes: *(A through E)* cylinders, balls, plates, cones, and hemispheres; *(F)* multisegmented electrode; *(G)* ring electrode; *(H)* differential-current-density electrode.

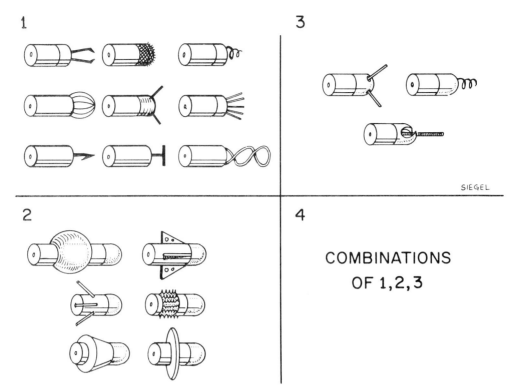

FIGURE 3-6. Various types of grasping elements incorporated on electrode tips. *(1)* In these designs, the electrode and the grasping element are one and the same. *(2)* These grasping elements are part of the lead rather than part of the electrode. *(3)* These grasping elements are independent of the electrode. *(4)* Various combinations of the above have been described.

Most electrodes are composed of platinum-iridium or stainless-steel alloys. But in order to avoid corrosion and polarization overpotentials, other materials have been used, such as carbon of various formulations. Some of these materials are almost nonpolarizing; moreover, the peak in stimulation threshold that normally occurs in 14 to 21 days is less obvious, and the chronic stimulation thresholds tend to be low. Platinum-iridium is still the standard with which all other electrode materials are compared.

In order to reduce the incidence of pervenous-electrode malposition (dislodgments and perforations), various bumps, baskets, whiskers, screws, and prongs have been added to the tip of the lead (Fig. 3-6). Sometimes the grasping element is active electrically, although this has not been considered a desirable combination because it increases the electrode surface area. In actual experience with leads of this type, late threshold elevation has been rare. The long-term durability of such a combination is as good as that of any other design, if not better. Leads are now conveniently categorized as grasping and nongrasping. With rare exceptions, modern leads tend to have some means of fixation, or at least of stabilizing the tip position.

A problem common to all leads with grasping or stabilizing mechanisms is difficulty in extracting the leads once they become affixed to the heart, and to the venous endothelial surfaces, by a fibrous tissue capsule. Fixation occurs where the lead makes contact with valves as well as with the venous conduits. Thus, once fibrous fixation has occurred, entrapment of the wide tip in the fibrous sheath may make it difficult or impossible to remove the lead. Although the body can tolerate inert foreign material fairly well, it cannot tolerate an infected foreign body. If infection should occur, it then would be essential to extract the lead. Therefore, a new lead that would be stable in its intracardiac position and, at the same time, easily removable is much to be desired.

The following chapters, a list of connector sizes for various pacemaker models and a catalogue of the leads and electrodes produced by today's manufacturers, should give the reader the information needed to select the appropriate lead for the clinical situation at hand.

CHAPTER **4**

LIST OF CONNECTOR SIZES* FOR VARIOUS PACEMAKER MODELS

Victor Parsonnet, M.D., Alan D. Bernstein, Eng.Sc.D., and Ralph Gallagher

UNIPOLAR, 5.0 mm

	Single-Chamber	Dual-Chamber
Biotronik	All models with "A" suffixes	
Cardiac Control Systems, Inc.	105	501
Cardiac Pacemakers, Inc.		910
Cook Pacemaker Corp.	331T	400
Coratomic, Inc.		Pulsar-1
Cordis Corp.		233G, 233GL
Intermedics, Inc.		263-01, 271-03, 283-01
Medtronic, Inc.	2443, 5923, 5927, 5941, 5967, 5973, 5983, 5985, 5989, 5995, 5995AP, 5997, 8403, 8423	5993SX, 7000, 7000A, 7100, 7100E, 7005
Pacesetter Systems, Inc.	241	223, 273, 275, 277, 283, 285
Telectronics	147, 155, 158B, 174, 274, 5281, 5281B	2251, 2291

---

* Arranged by (1) polarity, (2) connector size in mm, (3) single-chamber vs. dual-chamber, (4) manufacturer.

UNIPOLAR, 6.0 mm

	Single-Chamber	Dual-Chamber
Biotronik	All models with "B" suffixes	
Cardiac Pacemakers, Inc.	301, 501, 502, 503, 504, 505, 507, 508, 520, 521, 522, 523, 525, 530, 531, 702, 703	
Cook Pacemaker Corp.	215, 327D, 327T	
Coratomic, Inc.	VX5-105, C-101-P, Ovalith-920	
Cordis Corp.	334A, 336A, 337A, 402A, 402B	233F, 233GR, 415A
Intermedics, Inc.	253-01, 253-07, 253-19, 253-21	
Medtronic, Inc.		7005C
Pacesetter Systems, Inc.	225, 261	
Siemens-Elema	659, 668, 678, 688, 718	674
Telectronics	147, 155, 158B, 174, 5281, 5281B	2291

BIPOLAR, BIFURCATED 5.0 mm

	Single-Chamber	*Dual-Chamber*
Biotronik	All models with "ABP" suffixes	
Cardiac Pacemakers, Inc.	401, 601, 602, 603, 604, 605, 607, 608, 620, 621, 622, 623, 625, 630, 631, 802, 803	
Cook Pacemaker Corp.	216, 329T, 332T	
Coratomic, Inc.	VX5-205, Ovalith-920BP	
Cordis Corp.	336B, 402C	233F, 233GR, 415A
Intermedics, Inc.	254-07, 254-18, 262-01	
Medtronic, Inc.	5992, 5926, 5940, 5966, 5972, 5976, 5984, 5988, 5994, 5994AP, 5996, 8402, 8422	5992
Pacesetter Systems, Inc.	226, 242, 262	
Siemens-Elema	668B, 678B, 718B	
Telectronics	247, 2551, 4151, 4171, 4172, 5282	

BIPOLAR, IN-LINE, 3.2 mm

	Single-Chamber	Dual-Chamber
Cardiac Pacemakers, Inc.		925
Coratomic, Inc.	VX5-305	
Cordis Corp.		418A (ventricular lead only)
Medtronic, Inc.	5968, 5984LP, 8400, 8420	7006, 7008
Siemens-Elema	688L	
Telectronics	258, 5282A	

BIPOLAR, IN-LINE, 6.0 mm

	Single-Chamber	Dual-Chamber
Cordis Corp.	336A, 402A, 402B	415A (ventricular lead only)
Intermedics, Inc.	254-20	284-02

CHAPTER 5

LEAD ATLAS*

Victor Parsonnet, M.D., Alan D. Bernstein, Eng.Sc.D., and Ralph Gallagher

TABLE OF CONTENTS—LEADS

MANUFACTURER	MODEL	PAGE
Biotronic	DFH	S-149
	DJ	S-150
	D2K	S-151
	DN	S-152
	DYC	S-153
Cardiac Control Systems, Inc.	SV-101, SV-105	S-154
	SJ-103	S-155
	AV-102	S-156
Cardiac Pacemakers, Inc.	4266	S-157
Cordis Corp.	329-158P	S-158
	329-258	S-159
	329-259	S-160
	329-748P	S-161
	325-352, 325-342	S-162
Intermedics, Inc.	471-07	S-163
	471-09	S-164
	473-03	S-165
	476-03	S-166
	476-04	S-167
	479-01	S-168
	480-01	S-169
	483-03, 483-04	S-170
	486-01	S-171
	487-05	S-172

---

* Arranged alphabetically by manufacturer and secondarily by number when leads have model numbers.

MANUFACTURER	MODEL	PAGE
Intermedics, Inc.	492-01	S-173
	493-03	S-174
	493-05	S-175
Medtronic, Inc.	4003	S-176
	4011	S-177
	4012	S-178
	4503	S-179
	4511	S-180
	4512	S-181
	5061	S-182
	5062	S-183
	6912	S-184
Pacesetter Systems, Inc.	816	S-185
	820	S-186
	850	S-187
	851	S-188
	853	S-189
	865, 867	S-190
	866	S-191
	869	S-192
Siemens-Elema	402S	S-193
	404B	S-194
	411S	S-195
	412S	S-196
	415S	S-197

BIOTRONIK

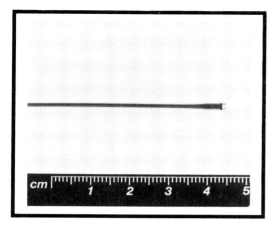 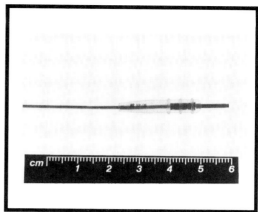

1. **IDENTIFICATION**
   Lead Model Number: DFH
   Special Name:

2. **GENERAL DESCRIPTION**
   Intended Use: pervenous
   Designed for: right atrium

3. **ELECTRODES**

	Electrode #1 (most distal)	Electrode #2 (next proximal)	Electrode #3 (next proximal)
Shape:	blunt cylinder with opposing hooks		
Surface Area:	12.0 mm²		
Material:	elgiloy		

   Remarks: Due to opposing hooks on tip, lead is passed pervenously with a counterclock-wise rotation, and anchored with a clockwise rotation.

4. **FIXATION MECHANISM:**   opposing hooks, depth of penetration = 0.9 mm

5. **WIRE**
   Configuration: quadrifilar helical coil
   Material: MP35N nickel alloy
   Insulation: Silastic
   Diameter of Shaft: 1.5 mm (4.5 FR)
   Maximum Insertion Diameter: 2.0 mm (6.0 FR)
   Length Option: 60 cm (custom length on request)
   Splice Kit Available: yes
   Lead Resistance: 1 ohm/cm
   Other Special Characteristics:

6. **CONNECTOR**
   Type: pin with setscrew
   Interconnection to Other Manufacturers without Adapter: 5- or 6-mm connectors on request

   Adapter Available: yes
   Extension Kit Available: yes
   New Connector Available: yes
   Conductor Material: stainless steel
   Metals Compatible with Other Manufacturers' Connectors: yes
   Special Features:

BIOTRONIK

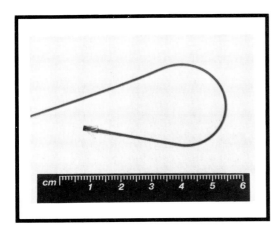 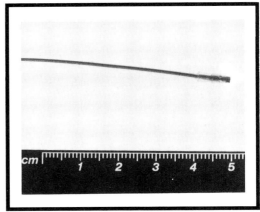

1. **IDENTIFICATION**
   Lead Model Number: DJ
   Special Name:

2. **GENERAL DESCRIPTION**
   Intended Use: pervenous
   Designed for: right atrial appendage

3. **ELECTRODES**

	Electrode #1 (most distal)	Electrode #2 (next proximal)	Electrode #3 (next proximal)
Shape:	blunt cylinder		
Surface Area:	10.0 mm²		
Material:	elgiloy		

   Remarks: "J" curve for positional stability

4. **FIXATION MECHANISM:**   tines

5. **WIRE**
   Configuration: helical coil (bifilar or quadrifilar)
   Material: MP35N nickel alloy
   Insulation: Silastic
   Diameter of Shaft: 1.5 mm (4.5 FR)
   Maximum Insertion Diameter: 3.0 mm (9.0 FR)
   Length Option: 60, 85 cm (custom length on request)
   Splice Kit Available: yes
   Lead Resistance: 1 ohm/cm
   Other Special Characteristics: "J" curve for positional stability

6. **CONNECTOR**
   Type: pin with setscrew
   Interconnection to Other Manufacturers without Adapter: 5- or 6-mm connectors on request

   Adapter Available: yes
   Extension Kit Available: yes
   New Connector Available: yes
   Conductor Material: stainless steel
   Metals Compatible with Other Manufacturers' Connectors: yes
   Special Features:

BIOTRONIK

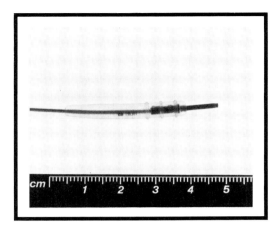 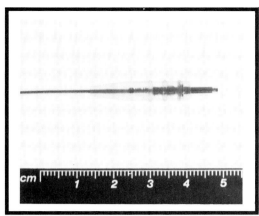

1. **IDENTIFICATION**
   Lead Model Number: D2K
   Special Name:

2. **GENERAL DESCRIPTION**
   Intended Use: pervenous
   Designed for: right ventricle

3. **ELECTRODES**

	Electrode #1 (most distal)	Electrode #2 (next proximal)	Electrode #3 (next proximal)
Shape:	blunt cylinder		
Surface Area:	10.0 mm²		
Material:	elgiloy		

   Remarks:

4. **FIXATION MECHANISM:**   double flange

5. **WIRE**
   Configuration: quadrifilar helical coil
   Material: MP35N nickel alloy
   Insulation: Silastic
   Diameter of Shaft: 1.5 mm (4.5 FR)
   Maximum Insertion Diameter: 3.0 mm (9.0 FR)
   Length Option: 60 cm (custom length on request)
   Splice Kit Available: yes
   Lead Resistance: 1 ohm/cm
   Other Special Characteristics:

6. **CONNECTOR**
   Type: pin with setscrew
   Interconnection to Other Manufacturers without Adapter: 5- or 6-mm connectors on request

   Adapter Available: yes
   Extension Kit Available: yes
   New Connector Available: yes
   Conductor Material: stainless steel
   Metals Compatible with Other Manufacturers' Connectors: yes
   Special Features:

BIOTRONIK

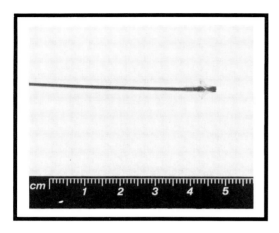
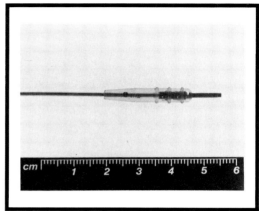

1. **IDENTIFICATION**
   Lead Model Number: DN
   Special Name:

2. **GENERAL DESCRIPTION**
   Intended Use: pervenous
   Designed for: right ventricle

3. **ELECTRODES**

	Electrode #1 (most distal)	Electrode #2 (next proximal)	Electrode #3 (next proximal)
Shape:	blunt cylinder		
Surface Area:	10.0 mm²		
Material:	elgiloy		

   Remarks:

4. **FIXATION MECHANISM:**   tines

5. **WIRE**
   Configuration: helical coil (bifilar or quadrifilar)
   Material: MP35N nickel alloy
   Insulation: Silastic
   Diameter of Shaft: 1.5 mm (4.5 FR)
   Maximum Insertion Diameter: 3.0 mm (9.0 FR)
   Length Option: 60, 85 cm (custom length on request)
   Splice Kit Available: yes
   Lead Resistance: 1 ohm/cm
   Other Special Characteristics:

6. **CONNECTOR**
   Type: pin with setscrew
   Interconnection to Other Manufacturers without Adapter: 5- or 6-mm connectors on request

   Adapter Available: yes
   Extension Kit Available: yes
   New Connector Available: yes
   Conductor Material: stainless steel
   Metals Compatible with Other Manufacturers' Connectors: yes
   Special Features:

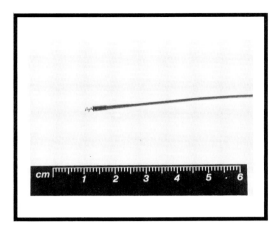
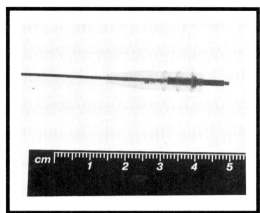

1. **IDENTIFICATION**
   Lead Model Number: DYC
   Special Name:

2. **GENERAL DESCRIPTION**
   Intended Use: pervenous
   Designed for: right ventricle

3. **ELECTRODES**

	Electrode #1 (most distal)	Electrode #2 (next proximal)	Electrode #3 (next proximal)
Shape:	screw-helix		
Surface Area:	13.0 mm²		
Material:	elgiloy		

   Remarks: Lead is passed transvenously with a counterclockwise rotation and anchored
               with a clockwise rotation. Depth of penetration = 2.5 mm

4. **FIXATION MECHANISM:**   screw-helix

5. **WIRE**
   Configuration: quadrifilar helical coil
   Material: MP35N nickel alloy
   Insulation: Silastic
   Diameter of Shaft: 1.5 mm (4.5 FR)
   Maximum Insertion Diameter: 2.0 mm (6.0 FR)
   Length Option: 60 cm (custom length on request)
   Splice Kit Available: yes
   Lead Resistance: 1 ohm/cm
   Other Special Characteristics:

6. **CONNECTOR**
   Type: pin with setscrew
   Interconnection to Other Manufacturers without Adapter: 5- or 6-mm connectors on request
   Adapter Available: yes
   Extension Kit Available: yes
   New Connector Available: yes
   Conductor Material: stainless steel
   Metals Compatible with Other Manufacturers' Connectors: yes
   Special Features:

CARDIAC CONTROL SYSTEMS, INC.

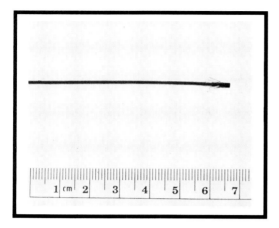 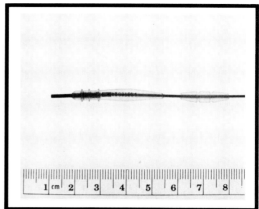

1. **IDENTIFICATION**
   Lead Model Number: SV-101, SV-105
   Special Name:

2. **GENERAL DESCRIPTION**
   Intended Use: pervenous
   Designed for: right ventricle

3. **ELECTRODES**

	Electrode #1 (most distal)	Electrode #2 (next proximal)	Electrode #3 (next proximal)
Shape:	blunt cylinder		
Surface Area:	11.0 mm²		
Material:	platinum-iridium		

   Remarks:

4. **FIXATION MECHANISM:**   tines

5. **WIRE**
   Configuration: helical coil
   Material: MP35N nickel alloy
   Insulation: polyurethane
   Diameter of Shaft: 1.4 mm (4.2 FR)
   Maximum Insertion Diameter: 2.9 mm (8.7 FR)
   Length Option: 56 cm (SV-101), 50 cm (SV-105)
   Splice Kit Available: no
   Lead Resistance: 48 ohms (SV-101), 42.5 ohms (SV-105)
   Other Special Characteristics:

6. **CONNECTOR**
   Type: pin with setscrew
   Interconnection to Other Manufacturers without Adapter: other 5-mm connectors

   Adapter Available: no
   Extension Kit Available: no
   New Connector Available: yes
   Conductor Material: 316L stainless steel
   Metals Compatible with Other Manufacturers' Connectors: yes
   Special Features:

CARDIAC CONTROL SYSTEMS, INC.

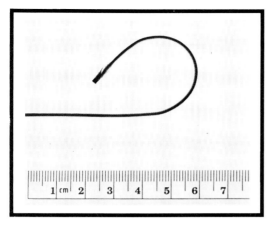
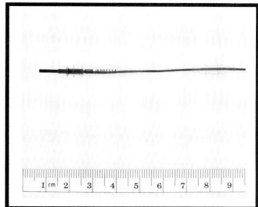

1. **IDENTIFICATION**
   Lead Model Number: SJ-103
   Special Name:

2. **GENERAL DESCRIPTION**
   Intended Use: pervenous
   Designed for: right atrial appendage

3. **ELECTRODE**

	Electrode #1 (most distal)	Electrode #2 (next proximal)	Electrode #3 (next proximal)
Shape:	blunt cylinder		
Surface Area:	11.0 mm^2		
Material:	platinum-iridium		
Remarks:			

4. **FIXATION MECHANISM:**   tines

5. **WIRE**
   Configuration: helical coil
   Material: MP35N nickel alloy
   Insulation: polyurethane
   Diameter of Shaft: 1.4 mm (4.2 FR)
   Maximum Insertion Diameter: 2.9 mm (8.7 FR)
   Length Option: 48 cm
   Splice Kit Available: no
   Lead Resistance: 32 ohms
   Other Special Characteristics: "J" curve for positional stability

6. **CONNECTOR**
   Type: pin with setscrew
   Interconnection to Other Manufacturers without Adapter: other 5-mm connectors

   Adapter Available: no
   Extension Kit Available: no
   New Connector Available: yes
   Conductor Material: 316L stainless steel
   Metals Compatible with Other Manufacturers' Connectors: yes
   Special Features:

CARDIAC CONTROL SYSTEMS, INC.

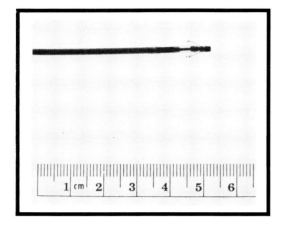
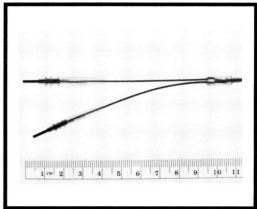

1. **IDENTIFICATION**
   Lead Model Number: AV-102
   Special Name: AV Data Lead

2. **GENERAL DESCRIPTION**
   Intended Use: pervenous
   Designed for: right ventricle

3. **ELECTRODES**

	Electrode #1 (most distal)	Electrode #2 (next proximal)	Electrode #3 (next proximal)
Shape:	blunt cylinder	ring	ring
Surface Area:	11.0 mm²	28.0 mm²	28.0 mm²
Material:	platinum-iridium	platinum-iridium	platinum-iridium (not shown)

   Remarks: Distal tip electrode used for unipolar ventricular pacing and sensing. Proximal ring electrodes provide an atrioventricular electrogram via programmer telemetry.

4. **FIXATION MECHANISM:**   tines

5. **WIRE**
   Configuration: helical coil
   Material: MP35N nickel alloy
   Insulation: polyurethane
   Diameter of Shaft: 2.1 mm (6.3 FR)
   Maximum Insertion Diameter: 2.9 mm (8.7 FR)
   Length Option: 56 cm
   Splice Kit Available: no
   Lead Resistance: 68 ohms to distal tip, 38 ohms to atrial ring, 48 ohms to ventricular ring
   Other Special Characteristics:

6. **CONNECTOR**
   Type: bifurcated pin with setscrew (distal electrode uses 5-mm connector; ring electrodes share a 4.5-mm connector)
   Interconnection to Other Manufacturers without Adapter: other 5-mm connectors (distal only; connector for A-V ring electrodes compatible with CCS pacemakers only)

   Adapter Available: no
   Extension Kit Available: no
   New Connector Available: yes
   Conductor Material: 316L stainless steel
   Metals Compatible with Other Manufacturers' Connectors: yes
   Special Features:

CARDIAC PACEMAKERS, INC.

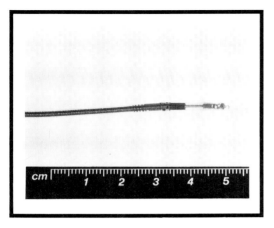 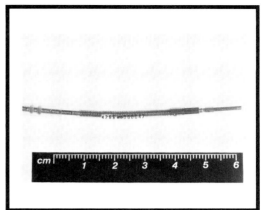

1. **IDENTIFICATION**
   Lead Model Number: 4266
   Special Name: Sentra

2. **GENERAL DESCRIPTION**
   Intended Use: pervenous
   Designed for: right atrium/right ventricle

3. **ELECTRODES**

	Electrode #1 (most distal)	Electrode #2 (next proximal)	Electrode #3 (next proximal)
Shape:	blunt ring	cylinder	
Surface Area:	10.0 mm^2	35 mm^2	
Material:	platinum-iridium	platinum-iridium	

   Remarks: Porous distal electrode enhances fixation. Distance between electrodes = 11 mm

4. **FIXATION MECHANISM:**   screw-helix—electrically isolated (1¾ turns penetration = 1.5 mm)

5. **WIRE**
   Configuration: coaxial helical coil (inner—bifilar, outer—quadrifilar)
   Material: MP35N nickel alloy
   Insulation: Silastic
   Diameter of Shaft: 2.2 mm (7.3 FR)
   Maximum Insertion Diameter: 3 mm (9.0 FR)
   Length Option: 52 cm
   Splice Kit Available: no
   Lead Resistance: 150 ohms bipolar
   Other Special Characteristics:

6. **CONNECTOR**
   Type: in-line low-profile pin with setscrew
   Interconnection to Other Manufacturers without Adapter: other in-line 3.2-mm connectors

   Adapter Available: yes
   Extension Kit Available: no
   New Connector Available: no
   Conductor Material: stainless steel
   Metals Compatible with Other Manufacturers' Connectors: yes
   Special Features:

CORDIS CORP.

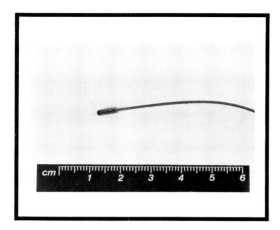
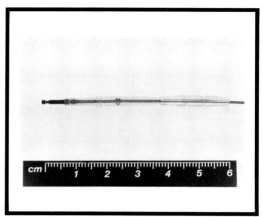

1. **IDENTIFICATION**
   Lead Model Number: 329-158P
   Special Name:

2. **GENERAL DESCRIPTION**
   Intended Use: pervenous
   Designed for: right ventricle

3. **ELECTRODES**

	Electrode #1 (most distal)	Electrode #2 (next proximal)	Electrode #3 (next proximal)
Shape:	hemispheric		
Surface Area:	8.0 mm²		
Material:	platinum-iridium		

   Remarks: porous surface enhances fixation

4. **FIXATION MECHANISM:**   3 fins

5. **WIRE**
   Configuration: quadrifilar helical coils
   Material: MP35N nickel alloy
   Insulation: polyurethane
   Diameter of Shaft: 1.25 mm (4.0 FR)
   Maximum Insertion Diameter: 2.6 mm (8 FR)
   Length Option: 58 cm
   Splice Kit Available: no
   Lead Resistance: 55 ohms
   Other Special Characteristics:

6. **CONNECTOR**
   Type: low profile pin with setscrew
   Interconnection to Other Manufacturers without Adapter: all 3.2-mm connectors

   Adapter Available: yes
   Extension Kit Available: yes
   New Connector Available: no
   Conductor Material: stainless steel
   Metals Compatible with Other Manufacturers' Connectors: yes
   Special Features:

CORDIS CORP.

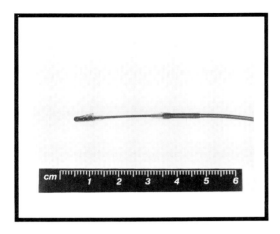 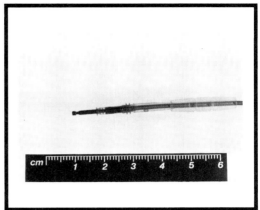

1. **IDENTIFICATION**
   Lead Model Number: 329-258
   Special Name:

2. **GENERAL DESCRIPTION**
   Intended Use: pervenous
   Designed for: right ventricle

3. **ELECTRODES**

	Electrode #1 (most distal)	Electrode #2 (next proximal)	Electrode #3 (next proximal)
Shape:	blunt cylinder	cylinder	
Surface Area:	8.0 mm^2	50.6 mm^2	
Material:	platinum-iridium	platinum-iridium	

   Remarks: porous surface on distal electrode enhances fixation. Distance between electrodes = 27 mm

4. **FIXATION MECHANISM:**   3 fins

5. **WIRE**
   Configuration: quadrifilar helical coils
   Material: MP35N nickel alloy
   Insulation: polyurethane
   Diameter of Shaft: 2.0 mm (6.0 FR)
   Maximum Insertion Diameter: 2.6 mm (8.0 FR)
   Length Option: 58 cm
   Splice Kit Available: no
   Lead Resistance: 130 ohms (bipolar)
   Other Special Characteristics:

6. **CONNECTOR**
   Type: in-line low-profile pin with setscrew
   Interconnection to Other Manufacturers without Adapter: all 3.2-mm connectors

   Adapter Available: yes
   Extension Kit Available: no
   New Connector Available: no
   Conductor Material: stainless steel
   Metals Compatible with Other Manufacturers' Connectors: yes
   Special Features:

CORDIS CORP.

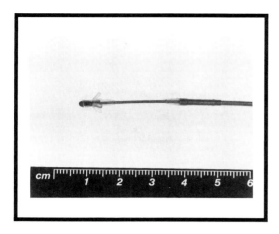 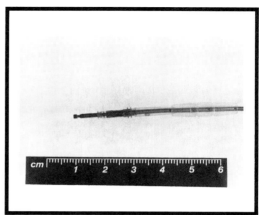

1. **IDENTIFICATION**
   Lead Model Number: 329-259
   Special Name:

2. **GENERAL DESCRIPTION**
   Intended Use: pervenous
   Designed for: right ventricle

3. **ELECTRODES**

	Electrode #1 (most distal)	Electrode #2 (next proximal)	Electrode #3 (next proximal)
Shape:	hemispheric	cylinder	
Surface Area:	8.0 mm^2	50.6 mm^2	
Material:	platinum-iridium	platinum-iridium	

   Remarks: porous surface on distal increases current density and enhances fixation. Distance between electrodes = 27 mm

4. **FIXATION MECHANISM:**   4 sawtooth tines

5. **WIRE**
   Configuration: quadrifilar helical coils
   Material: MP35N nickel alloy
   Insulation: polyurethane
   Diameter of Shaft: 2.0 mm (6.0 FR)
   Maximum Insertion Diameter: 3.5 mm (10.5 FR)
   Length Option: 58 cm
   Splice Kit Available: no
   Lead Resistance: 130 ohms (bipolar)
   Other Special Characteristics:

6. **CONNECTOR**
   Type: in-line low-profile pin with setscrew
   Interconnection to Other Manufacturers without Adapter: all 3.2-mm connectors

   Adapter Available: yes
   Extension Kit Available: yes
   New Connector Available: no
   Conductor Material: stainless steel
   Metals Compatible with Other Manufacturers' Connectors: yes
   Special Features:

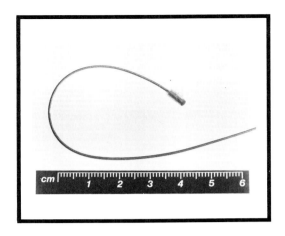 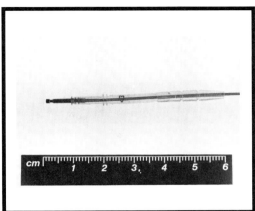

1. **IDENTIFICATION**
   Lead Model Number: 329-748P
   Special Name:

2. **GENERAL DESCRIPTION**
   Intended Use: pervenous
   Designed for: right atrial appendage

3. **ELECTRODES**

	Electrode #1 (most distal)	Electrode #2 (next proximal)	Electrode #3 (next proximal)
Shape:	blunt cylinder		
Surface Area:	8.8 mm^2		
Material:	platinum-iridium		

   Remarks: porous surface enhances fixation

4. **FIXATION MECHANISM:**   2 sawtooth tines

5. **WIRE**
   Configuration: quadrifilar helical coils
   Material: MP35N nickel alloy
   Insulation: polyurethane
   Diameter of Shaft: 1.5 mm (4.5 FR)
   Maximum Insertion Diameter: 3.5 mm (10.5 FR)
   Length Option: 48 cm
   Splice Kit Available: yes
   Lead Resistance: 80 ohms
   Other Special Characteristics: "J" curve for positional stability

6. **CONNECTOR**
   Type: low-profile pin with setscrew
   Interconnection to Other Manufacturers without Adapter: all 3.2-mm connectors

   Adapter Available: yes
   Extension Kit Available: yes
   New Connector Available: yes
   Conductor Material: stainless steel
   Metals Compatible with Other Manufacturers' Connectors: yes
   Special Features:

CORDIS CORP.

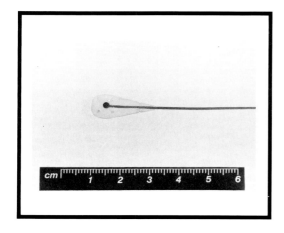 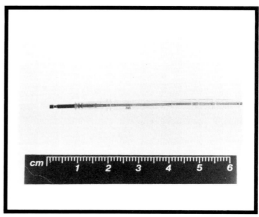

1. **IDENTIFICATION**
   Lead Model Number: 325–352, 325–342
   Special Name:

2. **GENERAL DESCRIPTION**
   Intended Use: myocardial
   Designed for: right/left ventricle

3. **ELECTRODES**

	Electrode #1 (most distal)	Electrode #2 (next proximal)	Electrode #2 (next proximal)
Shape:	disk		
Surface Area:	6.1 mm²		
Material:	platinum-iridium		

   Remarks: porous surface on distal electrode reduces chronic pacing thresholds.

4. **FIXATION MECHANISM:**   sutures

5. **WIRE**
   Configuration: quadrifilar helical coils
   Material: MP35N nickel alloy
   Insulation: polyurethane
   Diameter of Shaft: 1.25 mm (3.9 FR)
   Maximum Insertion Diameter: N/A
   Length Option: 52 cm
   Splice Kit Available: no
   Lead Resistance: 550 ohms
   Other Special Characteristics:

6. **CONNECTOR**
   Type: low-profile pin with setscrew
   Interconnection to Other Manufacturers without Adapter: other 3.2-mm connectors

   Adapter Available: yes
   Extension Kit Available: yes
   New Connector Available: yes
   Conductor Material: stainless steel
   Metals Compatible with Other Manufacturers' Connectors: yes
   Special Features: 325–452 is supplied with a temporary extension lead for temporary pacing applications.

INTERMEDICS, INC.

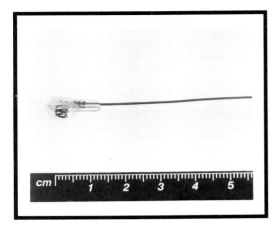 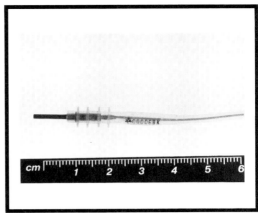

1. **IDENTIFICATION**
   Lead Model Number: 471–07
   Special Name:

2. **GENERAL DESCRIPTION**
   Intended Use: myocardial
   Designed for: right/left ventricle

3. **ELECTRODES**

	Electrode #1 (most distal)	Electrode #2 (next proximal)	Electrode #3 (next proximal)
Shape:	2-turn screw helix		
Surface Area:	8.0 mm²		
Material:	platinum-iridium		

   Remarks: maximum electrode penetration = 3.4 mm

4. **FIXATION MECHANISM:**   polyester mesh

5. **WIRE**
   Configuration: trifilar helical coils
   Material: nickel-cobalt alloy
   Insulation: Silastic
   Diameter of Shaft: 1.5 mm (4.5 FR)
   Maximum Insertion Diameter:
   Length Option: 35 cm
   Splice Kit Available: yes
   Lead Resistance: 40 ohms
   Other Special Characteristics:

6. **CONNECTOR**
   Type: pin with setscrew
   Interconnection to Other Manufacturers without Adapter: all 5- or 6-mm connectors

   Adapter Available: yes
   Extension Kit Available: yes
   New Connector Available: yes
   Conductor Material: 316 stainless steel
   Metals Compatible with Other Manufacturers' Connectors: yes
   Special Features:

INTERMEDICS, INC.

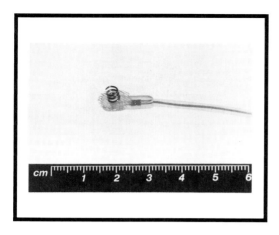 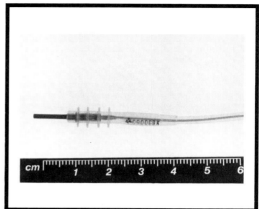

1. **IDENTIFICATION**
   Lead Model Number: 471–09
   Special Name:

2. **GENERAL DESCRIPTION**
   Intended Use: myocardial
   Designed for: right/left ventricle

3. **ELECTRODES**

	Electrode #1 (most distal)	Electrode #2 (next proximal)	Electrode #3 (next proximal)
Shape:	3-turn screw-helix		
Surface Area:	8.0 mm²		
Material:	platinum-iridium		

   Remarks: maximum electrode penetration = 5.0 mm

4. **FIXATION MECHANISM:**   polyester mesh

5. **WIRE**
   Configuration: trifilar helical coils
   Material: nickel cobalt alloy
   Insulation: Silastic
   Diameter of Shaft: 2.5 mm (7.5 FR)
   Maximum Insertion Diameter:
   Length Option: 35 cm
   Splice Kit Available: yes
   Lead Resistance: 40 ohms
   Other Special Characteristics:

6. **CONNECTOR**
   Type: pin with setscrew
   Interconnection to Other Manufacturers without Adapter: all 5- or 6-mm connectors

   Adapter Available: yes
   Extension Kit Available: yes
   New Connector Available: yes
   Conductor Material: 316 stainless steel
   Metals Compatible with Other Manufacturers' Connectors: yes
   Special Features:

INTERMEDICS, INC.

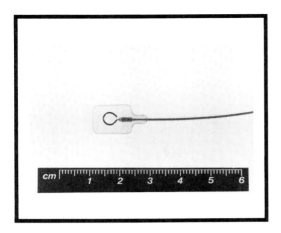 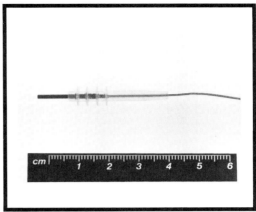

1. **IDENTIFICATION**
   Lead Model Number: 473-03
   Special Name:

2. **GENERAL DESCRIPTION**
   Intended Use: myocardial
   Designed for: right/left ventricle

3. **ELECTRODES**

	Electrode #1 (most distal)	Electrode #2 (next proximal)	Electrode #3 (next proximal)
Shape:	single loop		
Surface Area:	21 mm^2		
Material:	platinum-iridium		

   Remarks:

4. **FIXATION MECHANISM:**   sutures

5. **WIRE**
   Configuration: trifilar helical coils
   Material: nickel-cobalt alloy
   Insulation: polyurethane
   Diameter of Shaft: 1.3 mm (4.0 FR)
   Maximum Insertion Diameter: N/A
   Length Option: 45 cm
   Splice Kit Available: no
   Lead Resistance: 550 ohms
   Other Special Characteristics:

6. **CONNECTOR**
   Type: pin with setscrew
   Interconnection to Other Manufacturers without Adapter: all 5- or 6-mm connectors

   Adapter Available: yes
   Extension Kit Available: yes
   New Connector Available: yes
   Conductor Material: 316 stainless steel
   Metals Compatible with Other Manufacturers' Connectors: yes
   Special Features:

INTERMEDICS, INC.

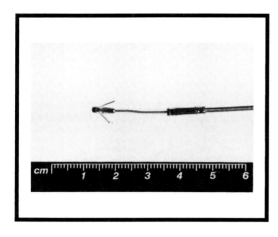 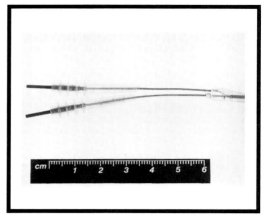

1. **IDENTIFICATION**
   Lead Model Number: 476-03
   Special Name:

2. **GENERAL DESCRIPTION**
   Intended Use: pervenous
   Designed for: right ventricle

3. **ELECTRODES**

	Electrode #1 (most distal)	Electrode #2 (next proximal)	Electrode #3 (next proximal)
Shape:	blunt ring	ring	
Surface Area:	10 mm²	50 mm²	
Material:	platinum-iridium	platinum-iridium	

   Remarks: distance between electrodes = 25.0 mm

4. **FIXATION MECHANISM:**   tines

5. **WIRE**
   Configuration: coaxial trifilar helical coils
   Material: nickel-cobalt alloy
   Insulation: polyurethane
   Diameter of Shaft: 2.0 mm (6.0 FR)
   Maximum Insertion Diameter: 3.0 mm (9.0 FR)
   Length Option: 40, 60 cm
   Splice Kit Available: no
   Lead Resistance: 70 ohms to distal electrode, 160 ohms to proximal electrode
   Other Special Characteristics:

6. **CONNECTOR**
   Type: bifurcated pin with setscrew
   Interconnection to Other Manufacturers without Adapter: all 5.0-mm connectors

   Adapter Available: yes
   Extension Kit Available: no
   New Connector Available: no
   Conductor Material: 316 stainless steel
   Metals Compatible with Other Manufacturers' Connectors: yes
   Special Features:

INTERMEDICS, INC.

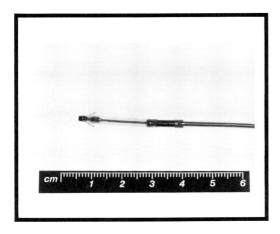 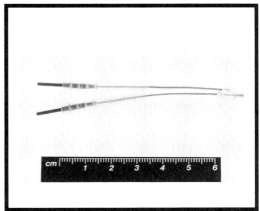

1. **IDENTIFICATION**
   Lead Model Number: 476-04
   Special Name:

2. **GENERAL DESCRIPTION**
   Intended Use: pervenous
   Designed for: right ventricle

3. **ELECTRODES**

	Electrode #1 (most distal)	Electrode #2 (next proximal)	Electrode #3 (next proximal)
Shape:	blunt ring	ring	
Surface Area:	10 mm²	50 mm²	
Material:	platinum-iridium	platinum-iridium	

   Remarks: distance between electrodes = 25 mm

4. **FIXATION MECHANISM:**   silicone-rubber tines

5. **WIRE**
   Configuration: trifilar helical coils
   Material: nickel cobalt alloy
   Insulation: Silastic
   Diameter of Shaft: 2.5 mm (7.5 FR)
   Maximum Insertion Diameter: 3.5 mm (10.5 FR)
   Length Option: 40, 60 cm
   Splice Kit Available: no
   Lead Resistance: 70 ohms to distal tip, 160 ohms to proximal ring
   Other Special Characteristics:

6. **CONNECTOR**
   Type: bifurcated pin with setscrew
   Interconnection to Other Manufacturers without Adapter: all 5- or 6-mm connectors

   Adapter Available: yes
   Extension Kit Available: no
   New Connector Available: no
   Conductor Material: 316 stainless steel
   Metals Compatible with Other Manufacturers' Connectors: yes
   Special Features:

INTERMEDICS, INC.

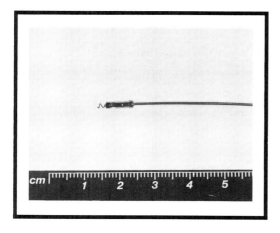 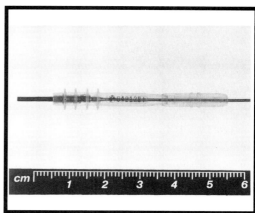

1. **IDENTIFICATION**
   Lead Model Number: 479-01
   Special Name:

2. **GENERAL DESCRIPTION**
   Intended Use: pervenous
   Designed for: right atrium or right ventricle

3. **ELECTRODES**

	Electrode #1 (most distal)	Electrode #2 (next proximal)	Electrode #3 (next proximal)
Shape:	ring		
Surface Area:	10.0 mm²		
Material:	platinum-iridium		
Remarks:			

4. **FIXATION MECHANISM:**   2-mm 1½-turn screw-in tip (electrically isolated with polymer coating)

5. **WIRE**
   Configuration: trifilar helical coils
   Material: nickel-cobalt alloy
   Insulation: polyurethane
   Diameter of Shaft: 1.7 mm (5.0 FR)
   Maximum Insertion Diameter: 2.2 mm (6.6 FR)
   Length Option: 40, 60 cm
   Splice Kit Available: no
   Lead Resistance: 750 ohms
   Other Special Characteristics:

6. **CONNECTOR**
   Type: pin with setscrew
   Interconnection to Other Manufacturers without Adapter: all 5- or 6-mm connectors

   Adapter Available: yes
   Extension Kit Available: yes
   New Connector Available: yes
   Conductor Material: 316 stainless steel
   Metals Compatible with Other Manufacturers' Connectors: yes
   Special Features:

INTERMEDICS, INC.

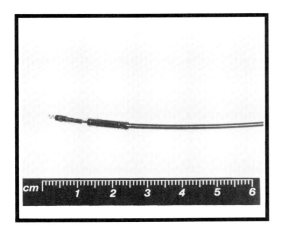 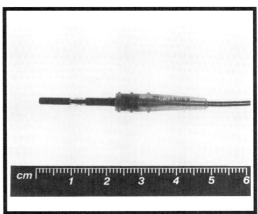

1. **IDENTIFICATION**
   Lead Model Number: 480-01
   Special Name:

2. **GENERAL DESCRIPTION**
   Intended Use: pervenous
   Designed for: right atrium or right ventricle

3. **ELECTRODES**

	Electrode #1 (most distal)	Electrode #2 (next proximal)	Electrode #3 (next proximal)
Shape:	blunt ring	ring	
Surface Area:	10.0 mm^2	50 mm^2	
Material:	platinum-iridium	platinum-iridium	

   Remarks:

4. **FIXATION MECHANISM:**   2-mm 1½-turn screw-in tip (electrically isolated with polymer coating)

5. **WIRE**
   Configuration: coaxial trifilar helical coils
   Material: nickel-cobalt alloy
   Insulation: polyurethane
   Diameter of Shaft: 2.0 mm (6.0 FR)
   Maximum Insertion Diameter: 2.7 mm (8.0 FR)
   Length Option: 40, 60 cm
   Splice Kit Available: no
   Lead Resistance: 70 ohms to distal electrode, 160 ohms to proximal electrode
   Other Special Characteristics:

6. **CONNECTOR**
   Type: in-line bipolar pin with setscrew
   Interconnection to Other Manufacturers without Adapter: all 5- or 6-mm connectors

   Adapter Available: yes
   Extension Kit Available: no
   New Connector Available: no
   Conductor Material: 316 stainless steel
   Metals Compatible with Other Manufacturers' Connectors: yes
   Special Features:

INTERMEDICS, INC.

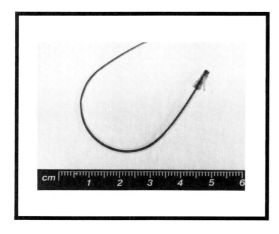 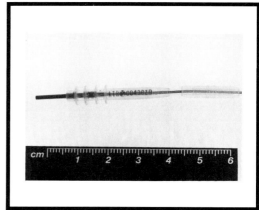

1. **IDENTIFICATION**
   Lead Model Number: 483-03, 483-04
   Special Name:

2. **GENERAL DESCRIPTION**
   Intended Use: pervenous
   Designed for: right atrial appendage

3. **ELECTRODES**

	Electrode #1 (most distal)	Electrode #2 (next proximal)	Electrode #3 (next proximal)
Shape:	blunt ring		
Surface Area:	10 mm²		
Material:	platinum-iridium		
Remarks:			

4. **FIXATION MECHANISM:**   tines

5. **WIRE**
   Configuration: trifilar helical coils
   Material: nickel-cobalt alloy
   Insulation: polyurethane
   Diameter of Shaft: 2.0 mm (6.0 FR)
   Maximum Insertion Diameter: 3.0 mm (9.0 FR)
   Length Option: 40, 60 cm
   Splice Kit Available: no
   Lead Resistance: 65 ohms
   Other Special Characteristics: "J" curve for positional stability (radius = 1.0 cm for 483-03, 1.5 cm for 483-04)

6. **CONNECTOR**
   Type: pin with setscrew
   Interconnection to Other Manufacturers without Adapter: all 5- or 6-mm connectors

   Adapter Available: yes
   Extension Kit Available: yes
   New Connector Available: yes
   Conductor Material: 316 stainless steel
   Metals Compatible with Other Manufacturers' Connectors: yes
   Special Features:

INTERMEDICS, INC.

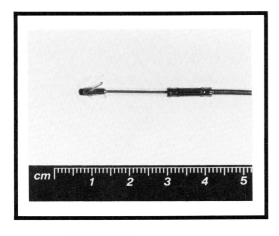 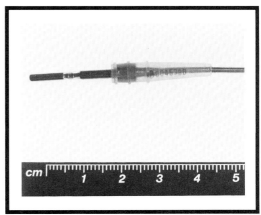

1. **IDENTIFICATION**
   Lead Model Number: 486–01
   Special Name:

2. **GENERAL DESCRIPTION**
   Intended Use: pervenous
   Designed for: right ventricle

3. **ELECTRODES**

	Electrode #1 (most distal)	Electrode #2 (next proximal)	Electrode #3 (next proximal)
Shape:	blunt ring	ring	
Surface Area:	10.0 mm^2	50.0 mm^2	
Material:	platinum-iridium	platinum-iridium	

   Remarks: distance between electrodes = 25.0 mm

4. **FIXATION MECHANISM:**   tines

5. **WIRE**
   Configuration: coaxial trifilar helical coils
   Material: nickel cobalt alloy
   Insulation: polyurethane
   Diameter of Shaft: 2.0 mm (6.0 FR)
   Maximum Insertion Diameter: 3.0 mm (9.0 FR)
   Length Option: 40, 60 cm
   Splice Kit Available: no
   Lead Resistance: 65 ohms to distal electrode, 150 ohms to proximal electrode
   Other Special Characteristics:

6. **CONNECTOR**
   Type: in-line bipolar pin with setscrew

   Interconnection to Other Manufacturers without Adapter: 6.0-mm connectors
   Adapter Available: yes
   Extension Kit Available: no
   New Connector Available: no
   Conductor Material: 316 stainless steel
   Metals Compatible with Other Manufacturers' Connectors: yes
   Special Features:

INTERMEDICS, INC.

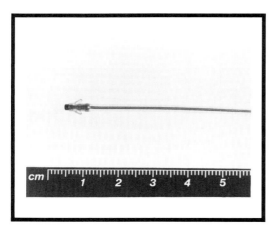 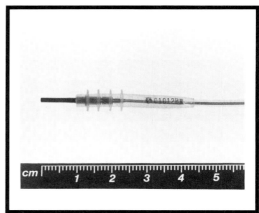

1. **IDENTIFICATION**
   Lead Model Number: 487-05
   Special Names:

2. **GENERAL DESCRIPTION**
   Intended Use: pervenous
   Designed for: right ventricle

3. **ELECTRODES**

	Electrode #1 (most distal)	Electrode #2 (next proximal)	Electrode #3 (next proximal)
Shape:	blunt ring		
Surface Area:	10 mm²		
Material:	platinum-iridium		

   Remarks:

4. **FIXATION MECHANISM:**   tines

5. **WIRE**
   Configuration: trifilar helical coils
   Material: nickel-cobalt alloy
   Insulation: Silastic
   Diameter of Shaft: 2.0 mm (6.0 FR)
   Maximum Insertion Diameter: 3.3 mm (10.0 FR)
   Length Option: 40, 60 cm
   Splice Kit Available: yes
   Lead Resistance: 750 ohms
   Other Special Characteristics:

6. **CONNECTOR**
   Type: pin with setscrew
   Interconnection to Other Manufacturers without Adapter: all 5- or 6-mm connectors

   Adapter Available: yes
   Extension Kit Available: yes
   New Connector Available: yes
   Conductor Material: 316 stainless steel
   Metals Compatible with Other Manufacturers' Connectors: yes
   Special Features:

INTERMEDICS, INC.

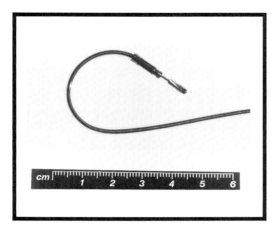 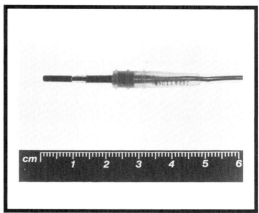

1. **IDENTIFICATION**
   Lead Model Number: 492-01
   Special Name:

2. **GENERAL DESCRIPTION**
   Intended Use: pervenous
   Designed for: right atrial appendage

3. **ELECTRODES**

	Electrode #1 (most distal)	Electrode #2 (next proximal)	Electrode #3 (next proximal)
Shape:	blunt ring	ring	
Surface Area:	10.0 mm^2	57.0 mm^2	
Material:	platinum-iridium	platinum-iridium	

   Remarks: distance between electrodes = 10.0 mm

4. **FIXATION MECHANISM:**   tines

5. **WIRE**
   Configuration: coaxial trifilar helical coils
   Material: nickel-cobalt alloy
   Insulation: polyurethane
   Diameter of Shaft: 2.7 mm (8.0 FR)
   Maximum Insertion Diameter: 3.0 mm (9.0 FR)
   Length Option: 54 cm
   Splice Kit Available: no
   Lead Resistance: 60 ohms to distal electrode, 135 ohms to proximal ring
   Other Special Characteristics: ''J'' curve for positional stability

6. **CONNECTOR**
   Type: in-line bipolar pin with setscrew
   Interconnection to Other Manufacturers without Adapter: 6-mm connectors

   Adapter Available: yes
   Extension Kit Available: no
   New Connector Available: no
   Conductor Material: 316 stainless steel
   Metals Compatible with Other Manufacturers' Connectors: yes
   Special Features:

INTERMEDICS, INC.

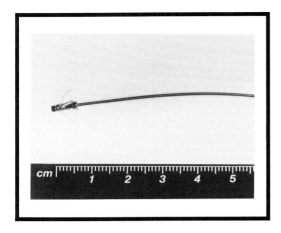 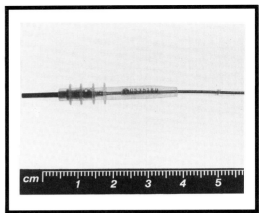

1. **IDENTIFICATION**
   Lead Model Number: 493-03
   Special Name:

2. **GENERAL DESCRIPTION**
   Intended Use: pervenous
   Designed for: right ventricle

3. **ELECTRODES**

	Electrode #1 (most distal)	Electrode #2 (next proximal)	Electrode #3 (next proximal)
Shape:	blunt ring		
Surface Area:	10 mm²		
Material:	platinum-iridium		
Remarks:			

4. **FIXATION MECHANISM:**   tines

5. **WIRE**
   Configuration: trifilar helical coils
   Material: nickel-cobalt alloy
   Insulation: polyurethane
   Diameter of Shaft: 1.3 mm (5.0 FR)
   Maximum Insertion Diameter: 3.0 mm (9.0 FR)
   Length Option: 40, 60 cm
   Splice Kit Available: no
   Lead Resistance: 75 ohms
   Other Special Characteristics:

6. **CONNECTOR**
   Type: pin with setscrew
   Interconnection to Other Manufacturers without Adapters: all 5- or 6-mm connectors

   Adapter Available: yes
   Extension Kit Available: yes
   New Connector Available: no
   Conductor Material: 316 stainless steel
   Metals Compatible with Other Manufacturers' Connectors: yes
   Special Features:

INTERMEDICS, INC.

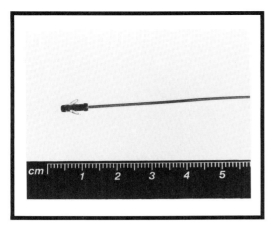 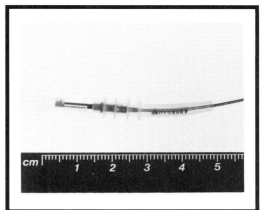

1. **IDENTIFICATION**
   Lead Model Number: 493-05
   Special Name: Bipore

2. **GENERAL DESCRIPTION**
   Intended Use: pervenous
   Designed for: right ventricle

3. **ELECTRODES**

	Electrode #1 (most distal)	Electrode #2 (next proximal)	Electrode #3 (next proximal)
Shape:	blunt cylinder		
Surface Area:	11 mm^2		
Material:	Biolite carbon porous titanium		

   Remarks:

4. **FIXATION MECHANISM:**   silicone tines

5. **WIRE**
   Configuration: trifilar helical coils
   Material: nickel-cobalt alloy
   Insulation: polyurethane
   Diameter of Shaft: 1.7 mm (5.0 FR)
   Maximum Insertion Diameter: 3.3 mm (10.0 FR)
   Length Option: 40, 60 cm
   Splice Kit Available: no
   Lead Resistance: 75 ohms
   Other Special Characteristics:

6. **CONNECTOR**
   Type: pin with setscrew
   Interconnection to Other Manufacturers without Adapter: all 5- or 6-mm connectors

   Adapter Available: yes
   Extension Kit Available: yes
   New Conductor Available: yes
   Conductor Material: 316 stainless steel
   Metals Compatible with Other Manufacturers' Connectors: yes
   Special Features:

MEDTRONIC, INC.

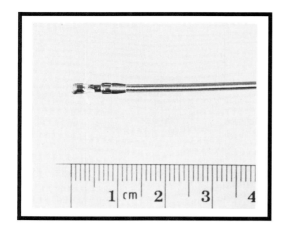 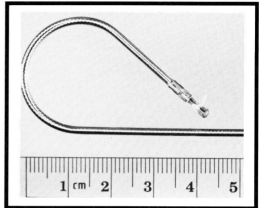

1. IDENTIFICATION
Lead Model Number: 4003
Special Name:

2. GENERAL DESCRIPTION
Intended Use: pervenous
Designed for: right ventricle

3. ELECTRODES

	Electrode #1 (most distal)	Electrode #2 (next proximal)	Electrode #3 (next proximal)
Shape:	porous hemispheric tip		
Surface Area:	8 mm²		
Material:	platinum-coated titanium		

Remarks: dexamethasone steroid elutes from tip to reduce tissue inflammation, thereby reducing threshold and threshold peaking

4. FIXATION MECHANISM: tines

5. WIRE
Configuration: helical coil
Material: MP35N nickel alloy
Insulation: polyurethane
Diameter of Shaft: 1.65 mm (4 FR)
Maximum Insertion Diameter: 3.0 mm (9 FR)
Length Option: 58 cm standard (20 to 110 cm available)
Splice Kit Available: no
Lead Resistance: less than or equal to 50 ohms
Other Special Characteristics:

6. CONNECTOR
Type: pin with setscrew
Interconnection to Other Manufacturers without Adapter: other 5-mm connectors

Adapter Available: yes
Extension Kit Available: yes
New Connector Available: yes
Conductor Material: 304 stainless steel
Metals Compatible with Other Manufacturers' Connectors: yes
Special Features:

MEDTRONIC, INC.

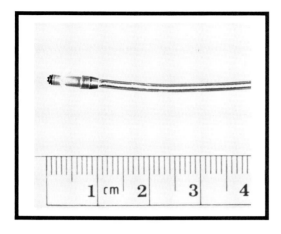 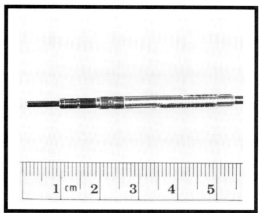

1. **IDENTIFICATION**
   Lead Model Number: 4011
   Special Name:

2. **GENERAL DESCRIPTION**
   Intended Use: pervenous
   Designed for: right ventricle

3. **ELECTRODES**

	Electrode #1 (most distal)	Electrode #2 (next proximal)	Electrode #3 (next proximal)
Shape:	hemispheric		
Surface Area:	8.4 mm²		
Material:	platinized platinum alloy		

   Remarks: two concentric grooves and platinized porous surface are designed to reduce polarization, and enhance fixation

4. **FIXATION MECHANISM:**   4 5.0-mm tines

5. **WIRE**
   Configuration: helical coil
   Material: MP35N nickel alloy
   Insulation: polyurethane
   Diameter of Shaft: 1.52 mm (4.6 FR)
   Maximum Insertion Diameter: 3.4 mm (10.4 FR)
   Length Option: 58 cm standard (20 to 110 cm available)
   Splice Kit Available: no
   Lead Resistance: 45 ohms (58 cm)
   Other Special Characteristics:

6. **CONNECTOR**
   Type: pin with setscrew
   Interconnection to Other Manufacturers without Adapter: other 5-mm connectors

   Adapter Available: yes
   Extension Kit Available: yes
   New Connector Available: yes
   Conductor Material: 304 stainless steel
   Metals Compatible with Other Manufacturers' Connectors: yes
   Special Features:

MEDTRONIC, INC.

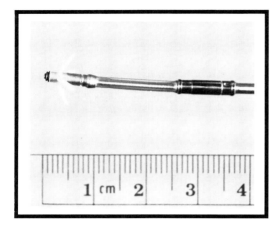 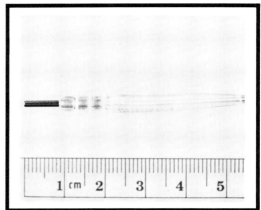

1. **IDENTIFICATION**
   Lead Model Number: 4012
   Special Name:

2. **GENERAL DESCRIPTION**
   Intended Use: pervenous
   Designed for: right ventricle

3. **ELECTRODES**

	Electrode #1 (most distal)	Electrode #2 (next proximal)	Electrode #3 (next proximal)
Shape:	hemispheric	ring	
Surface Area:	8.4 mm²	52 mm²	
Material:	platinized platinum alloy	platinum alloy	

   Remarks: two concentric grooves and platinized porous surface are designed to reduce polarization and enhance fixation. Distance between electrodes = 28 mm

4. **FIXATION MECHANISM:**   4 5.0-mm tines

5. **WIRE**
   Configuration: coaxial helical coil
   Material: MP35N nickel alloy
   Insulation: polyurethane
   Diameter of Shaft: 2.29 mm (6.9 FR)
   Maximum Insertion Diameter: 3.4 mm (10.4 FR)
   Length Option: 58 cm standard (20 to 110 cm available)
   Splice Kit Available: no
   Lead Resistance: 65 ohms (bipolar, 58 cm)
   Other Special Characteristics:

6. **CONNECTOR**
   Type: in-line low-profile pin with setscrew
   Interconnection to Other Manufacturers without Adapter: other 3.2-mm in-line connectors

   Adapter Available: yes
   Extension Kit Available: yes, with intermediate adapter
   New Connector Available: no
   Conductor Material: 304 stainless steel
   Metals Compatible with Other Manufacturers' Connectors: yes
   Special Features:

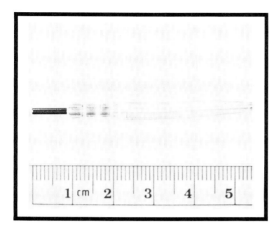 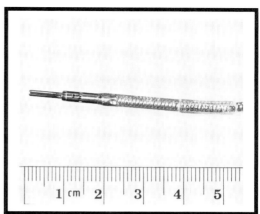

1. **IDENTIFICATION**
   Lead Model Number: 4503
   Special Name:

2. **GENERAL DESCRIPTION**
   Intended Use: pervenous
   Designed for: right atrium

3. **ELECTRODES**

	Electrode #1 (most distal)	Electrode #2 (next proximal)	Electrode #3 (next proximal)
Shape:	porous hemispheric tip		
Surface Area:	8 mm²		
Material:	platinum-coated titanium		

   Remarks: dexamethasone steroid elutes from tip to reduce tissue inflammation, thereby reducing threshold and threshold peaking

4. **FIXATION MECHANISM:**   tines

5. **WIRE**
   Configuration: helical coil
   Material: MP35N nickel alloy
   Insulation: polyurethane
   Diameter of Shaft: 1.65 mm (5 FR)
   Maximum Insertion Diameter: 3.0 mm (9 FR)
   Length Option: 58 cm standard (20 to 110 cm available)
   Splice Kit Available: no
   Lead Resistance: less than or equal to 50 ohms
   Other Special Characteristics: "J" curve for positional stability

6. **CONNECTOR**
   Type: pin with setscrew
   Interconnection to Other Manufacturers without Adapter: other 5-mm connectors

   Adapter Available: yes
   Extension Kit Available: no
   New Connector Available: yes
   Conductor Material: 304 stainless steel
   Metals Compatible with Other Manufacturers' Connectors: yes
   Special Features:

MEDTRONIC, INC.

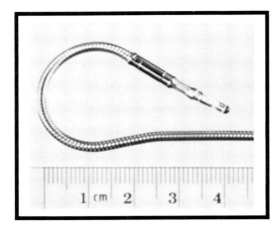 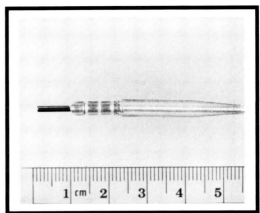

1. **IDENTIFICATION**
   Lead Model Number: 4511
   Special Name:

2. **GENERAL DESCRIPTION**
   Intended Use: pervenous
   Designed for: right atrial appendage

3. **ELECTRODES**

	Electrode #1 (most distal)	Electrode #2 (next proximal)	Electrode #3 (next proximal)
Shape:	hemispheric		
Surface Area:	8.4 mm^2		
Material:	platinized platinum alloy		

   Remarks: two concentric grooves and platinized porous surface designed to reduce polarization and enhance fixation

4. **FIXATION MECHANISM:**   3 5.0-mm tines

5. **WIRE**
   Configuration: coaxial helical coil
   Material: MP35N nickel alloy
   Insulation: polyurethane
   Diameter of Shaft: 1.98 mm (6.0 FR)
   Maximum Insertion Diameter: 3.4 mm (10.4 FR)
   Length Option: 53 cm standard (20 to 110 cm available)
   Splice Kit Available: no
   Lead Resistance: 11 ohms (53 cm)
   Other Special Characteristics: "J" curve for positional stability

6. **CONNECTOR**
   Type: pin with setscrew
   Interconnection to Other Manufacturers without Adapter: other 5-mm connectors

   Adapter Available: yes
   Extension Kit Available: yes
   New Connector Available: yes
   Conductor Material: 304 stainless steel
   Metals Compatible with Other Manufacturers' Connectors: yes
   Special Features:

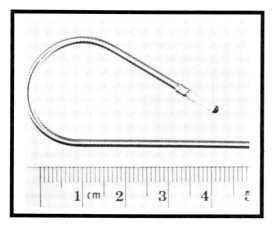
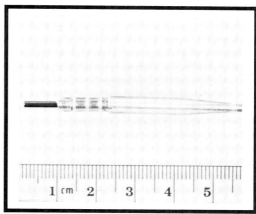

1. **IDENTIFICATION**
   Lead Model Number: 4512
   Special Name:

2. **GENERAL DESCRIPTION**
   Intended Use: pervenous
   Designed for: right atrial appendage

3. **ELECTRODES**

	Electrode #1 (most distal)	Electrode #2 (next proximal)	Electrode #3 (next proximal)
Shape:	hemispheric	ring	
Surface Area:	8.4 mm^2	52 mm^2	
Material:	platinized platinum alloy	platinum alloy	

   Remarks: two concentric grooves and platinized porous surface designed to reduce polarization and enhance fixation. Distance between electrodes = 17 mm

4. **FIXATION MECHANISM:**   3 5.0-mm tines

5. **WIRE**
   Configuration: coaxial helical coil
   Material: MP35N nickel alloy
   Insulation: polyurethane
   Diameter of Shaft: 2.46 mm (7.5 FR)
   Maximum Insertion Diameter: 3.4 mm (10.4 FR)
   Length Option: 53 cm standard (20 to 110 cm available)
   Splice Kit Available: no
   Lead Resistance: 63 ohms (bipolar, 53 cm)
   Other Special Characteristics: ''J'' curve for positional stability

6. **CONNECTOR**
   Type: in-line low-profile pin with setscrew
   Interconnection to Other Manufacturers without Adapter: other 3.2-mm in-line connectors

   Adapter Available: yes
   Extension Kit Available: yes, with intermediate adapter
   New Connector Available: no
   Conductor Material: 304 stainless steel
   Metals Compatible with Other Manufacturers' Connectors: yes
   Special Features:

MEDTRONIC, INC.

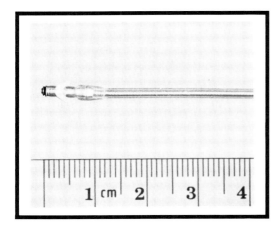 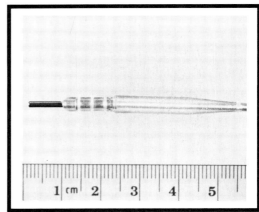

1. **IDENTIFICATION**
   Lead Model Number: 5061
   Special Name:

2. **GENERAL DESCRIPTION**
   Intended Use: pervenous
   Designed for: right ventricle

3. **ELECTRODES**

	Electrode #1 (most distal)	Electrode #2 (next proximal)	Electrode #3 (next proximal)
Shape:	hemispheric		
Surface Area:	8.4 mm^2		
Material:	platinized platinum alloy		

   Remarks: two concentric grooves and platinized porous surface are designed to reduce polarization and enhance fixation

4. **FIXATION MECHANISM:**   tines

5. **WIRE**
   Configuration: helical coil
   Material: MP35N nickel alloy
   Insulation: Silastic
   Diameter of Shaft: 2.16 mm (6.5 FR)
   Maximum Insertion Diameter: 3.8 mm (11.0 FR)
   Length Option: 58 cm standard (20 to 110 cm available)
   Splice Kit Available: no
   Lead Resistance: 45 ohms (58 cm)
   Other Special Characteristics:

6. **CONNECTOR**
   Type: pin with setscrew
   Interconnection to Other Manufacturers without Adapter: other 5-mm connectors

   Adapter Available: yes
   Extension Kit Available: yes
   New Connector Available: yes
   Conductor Material: 304 stainless steel
   Metals Compatible with Other Manufacturers' Connectors: yes
   Special Features:

MEDTRONIC, INC.

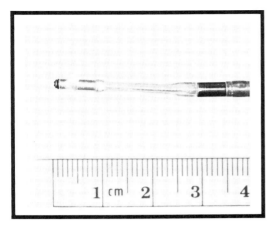 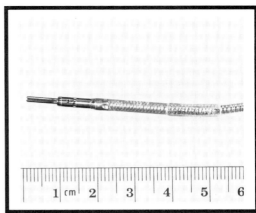

1. **IDENTIFICATION**
   Lead Model Number: 5062
   Special Name:

2. **GENERAL DESCRIPTION**
   Intended Use: pervenous
   Designed for: right ventricle

3. **ELECTRODES**

	Electrode #1 (most distal)	Electrode #2 (next proximal)	Electrode #3 (next proximal)
Shape:	hemispheric	ring	
Surface Area:	8.4 mm²	48 mm²	
Material:	platinized platinum alloy	platinum alloy	

   Remarks: two concentric grooves and platinized porous surface are designed to reduce polarization and enhance fixation

4. **FIXATION MECHANISM:**   4 5.0-mm tines

5. **WIRE**
   Configuration: coaxial helical coil
   Material: MP35N nickel alloy
   Insulation: Silastic
   Diameter of Shaft: 2.64 mm (8.0 FR)
   Maximum Insertion Diameter: 3.8 mm (11.0 FR)
   Length Option: 58 cm standard (20 to 110 cm available)
   Splice Kit Available: no
   Lead Resistance: 65 ohms (58 cm)
   Other Special Characteristics:

6. **CONNECTOR**
   Type: in-line low-profile pin with setscrew
   Interconnection to Other Manufacturers without Adapter: other 3.2-mm connectors

   Adapter Available: yes
   Extension Kit Available: yes, with an intermediate adapter
   New Connector Available: no
   Conductor Material: 304 stainless steel
   Metals Compatible with Other Manufacturers' Connectors: yes
   Special Features:

MEDTRONIC, INC.

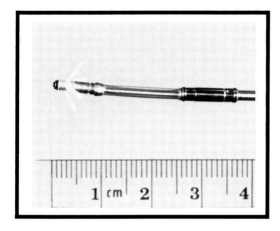 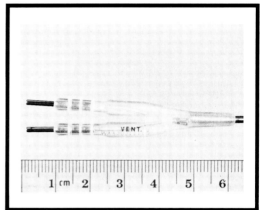

1. **IDENTIFICATION**
   Lead Model Number: 6912
   Special Name:

2. **GENERAL DESCRIPTION**
   Intended Use: pervenous
   Designed for: right ventricle

3. **ELECTRODES**

	Electrode #1 (most distal)	Electrode #2 (next proximal)	Electrode #3 (next proximal)
Shape:	hemispheric	ring	
Surface Area:	8.4 mm^2	52 mm^2	
Material:	platinized platinum alloy	platinum alloy	

   Remarks: two concentric grooves and platinized porous surface are designed to reduce polarization and enhance fixation

4. **FIXATION MECHANISM:**   tines

5. **WIRE**
   Configuration: coaxial helical coil
   Material: MP35N nickel alloy
   Insulation: polyurethane
   Diameter of Shaft: 2.29 mm (6.9 FR)
   Maximum Insertion Diameter: 3.4 mm (10.4 FR)
   Length Option: 58 cm standard (20 to 110 cm available)
   Splice Kit Available: no
   Lead Resistance: 65 ohms (58 cm)
   Other Special Characteristics:

6. **CONNECTOR**
   Type: bifurcated pin with setscrew
   Interconnection to Other Manufacturers without Adapter: other 5-mm connectors

   Adapter Available: yes
   Extension Kit Available: yes
   New Connector Available: yes
   Conductor Material: 304 stainless steel
   Metals Compatible with Other Manufacturers' Connectors: yes
   Special Features:

PACESETTER SYSTEMS, INC.

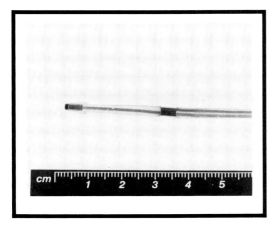
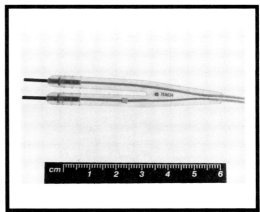

1. **IDENTIFICATION**
   Lead Model Number: 816
   Special Name:

2. **GENERAL DESCRIPTION**
   Intended Use: pervenous
   Designed for: right ventricle

3. **ELECTRODES**

	Electrode #1 (most distal)	Electrode #2 (next proximal)	Electrode #3 (next proximal)
Shape:	blunt cylinder	ring	
Surface Area:	10.0 mm²	48 mm²	
Material:	platinum-iridium	platinum-iridium	

   Remarks:

4. **FIXATION MECHANISM:**   flange

5. **WIRE**
   Configuration: unifilar helical coil
   Material: MP35N nickel alloy
   Insulation: Silastic
   Diameter of Shaft: 3.3 mm (10.0 FR)
   Maximum Insertion Diameter: 3.7 mm (11.0 FR)
   Length Option: 60, 85 cm
   Splice Kit Available: no
   Lead Resistance: 850 ohms (60 cm), 120 ohms (85 cm)
   Other Special Characteristics:

6. **CONNECTOR**
   Type: bifurcated pin with setscrew
   Interconnection to Other Manufacturers without Adapter: 5-mm connectors

   Adapter Available: yes
   Extension Kit Available: no
   New Connector Available: no
   Conductor Material: 316L stainless steel
   Metals Compatible with other Manufacturers' Connectors: yes
   Special Features:

PACESETTER SYSTEMS, INC.

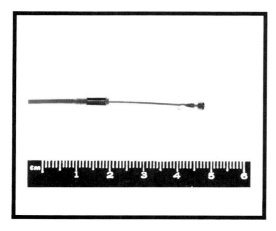
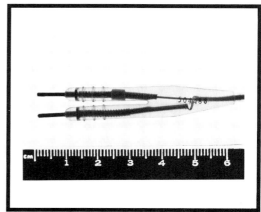

1. **IDENTIFICATION**
   Lead Model Number: 820
   Special Name:

2. **GENERAL DESCRIPTION**
   Intended Use: pervenous
   Designed for: right ventricle

3. **ELECTRODES**

	Electrode #1 (most distal	Electrode #2 (next proximal)	Electrode #3 (next proximal)
Shape:	blunt ring	ring	
Surface Area:	10.0 mm²	48.0 mm²	
Material:	platinum-iridium	platinum-iridium	

   Remarks:

4. **FIXATION MECHANISM:**   tines

5. **WIRE**
   Configuration: coaxial helical coil
   Material: MP35N nickel alloy
   Insulation: Silastic
   Diameter of Shaft: 2.9 mm (8.8 FR)
   Maximum Insertion Diameter: 3.3 mm (10 FR)
   Length Option: 52, 60, 85 cm
   Splice Kit Available: no
   Lead Resistance: distal—60 ohms (52 cm), 70 ohms (60 cm), 100 ohms (85 cm); proximal—
        30 ohms (52 cm), 35 ohms (60 cm), 50 ohms (85 cm)
   Other Special Characteristics:

6. **CONNECTOR**
   Type: bifurcated pin with setscrew
   Interconnection to Other Manufacturers without Adapter: other 5-mm connectors

   Adapter Available: yes
   Extension Kit Available: no
   New Connector Available: no
   Conductor Material: 316L stainless steel
   Metals Compatible with Other Manufacturers' Connectors:
   Special Features:

PACESETTER SYSTEMS, INC.

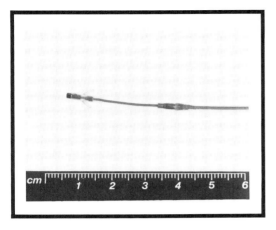 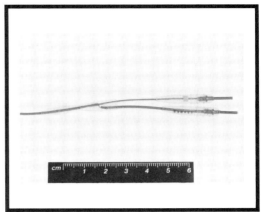

1. **IDENTIFICATION**
   Lead Model Number: 850
   Special Name:

2. **GENERAL DESCRIPTION**
   Intended Use: pervenous
   Designed for: right ventricle

3. **ELECTRODES**

	Electrode #1 (most distal)	Electrode #2 (next proximal)	Electrode #3 (next proximal)
Shape:	blunt ring	ring	
Surface Area:	8.0 mm²	48 mm²	
Material:	platinum-iridium	platinum-iridium	

   Remarks:

4. **FIXATION MECHANISM:**   tines

5. **WIRE**
   Configuration: coaxial helical coil (inner—trifilar, outer—quadrifilar)
   Material: MP35N nickel alloy
   Insulation: Silastic
   Diameter of Shaft: 1.7 mm (5.0 FR)
   Maximum Insertion Diameter: 3.0 mm (9.0 FR)
   Length Option: 60 cm
   Splice Kit Available: no
   Lead Resistance: 69 ohms each leg
   Other Special Characteristics:

6. **CONNECTOR**
   Type: bifurcated pin with setscrew
   Interconnection to Other Manufacturers without Adapter: all 5-mm connectors

   Adapter Available: yes
   Extension Kit Available: no
   New Connector Available: no
   Conductor Material: 316L stainless steel
   Metals Compatible with Other Manufacturers' Connectors: yes
   Special Features:

PACESETTER SYSTEMS, INC.

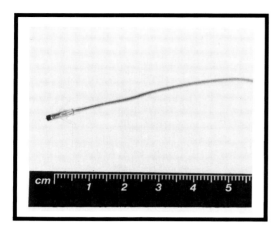 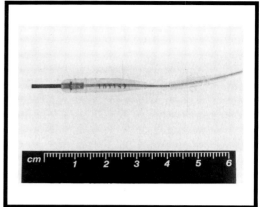

1. **IDENTIFICATION**
   Lead Model Number: 851
   Special Name:

2. **GENERAL DESCRIPTION**
   Intended Use: pervenous
   Designed for: right ventricle

3. **ELECTRODES**

	Electrode #1 (most distal)	Electrode #2 (next proximal)	Electrode #3 (next proximal)
Shape:	blunt ring		
Surface Area:	8.0 mm^2		
Material:	platinum-iridium		

   Remarks:

4. **FIXATION MECHANISM:**   tines

5. **WIRE**
   Configuration: trifilar helical coil
   Material: MP35N nickel alloy
   Insulation: Silastic
   Diameter of Shaft: 1.5 mm (4.5 FR)
   Maximum Insertion Diameter: 3.0 mm (9.0 FR)
   Length Option: 60 cm
   Splice Kit Available: no
   Lead Resistance: 50 ohms
   Other Special Characteristics: hydromer coating used to lower coefficient of friction

6. **CONNECTOR**
   Type: pin with setscrew
   Interconnection to Other Manufacturers without Adapter: 5-mm connectors

   Adapter Available: yes
   Extension Kit Available: no
   New Connector Available: yes
   Conductor Material: 316L stainless steel
   Metals Compatible with Other Manufacturers' Connectors: yes
   Special Features:

PACESETTER SYSTEMS, INC.

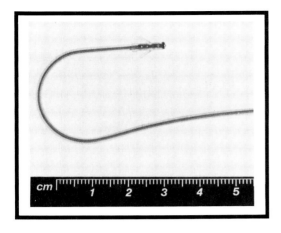 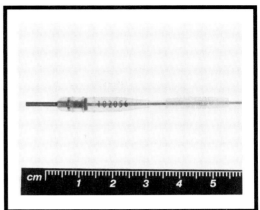

1. **IDENTIFICATION**
   Lead Model Number: 853
   Special Name:

2. **GENERAL DESCRIPTION**
   Intended Use: pervenous
   Designed for: right atrial appendage

3. **ELECTRODES**

	Electrode #1 (most distal)	Electrode #2 (next proximal)	Electrode #3 (next proximal)
Shape:	blunt ring		
Surface Area:	8.0 mm²		
Material:	platinum-iridium		
Remarks:			

4. **FIXATION MECHANISM:**   tines

5. **WIRE**
   Configuration: bifilar helical coil ("J" curve is unifilar)
   Material: MP35N nickel alloy
   Insulation: Silastic
   Diameter of Shaft: 1.8 mm (5.3 FR)
   Maximum Insertion Diameter: 3.3 mm (10.0 FR)
   Length Option: 52 cm
   Splice Kit Available: no
   Lead Resistance: 85 ohms
   Other Special Characteristics: hydromer coating used to lower coefficient of friction. "J" curve for positional stability.

6. **CONNECTOR**
   Type: pin with setscrew
   Interconnection to Other Manufacturers without Adapter: 5-mm connectors

   Adapter Available: yes
   Extension Kit Available: no
   New Connector Available: yes
   Conductor Material: 316L stainless steel
   Metals Compatible with Other Manufacturers' Connectors: yes
   Special Features:

PACESETTER SYSTEMS, INC.

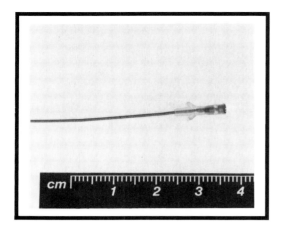 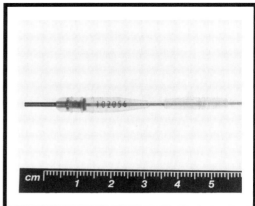

1. **IDENTIFICATION**
   Lead Model Number: 865, 867
   Special Name:

2. **GENERAL DESCRIPTION**
   Intended Use: transvenous
   Designed for: right ventricle

3. **ELECTRODES**

	Electrode #1 (most distal)	Electrode #2 (next proximal)	Electrode #3 (next proximal)
Shape:	blunt ring		
Surface Area:	8.0 mm²		
Material:	platinum-iridium		

   Remarks:

4. **FIXATION MECHANISM:**   tines

5. **WIRE**
   Configuration: trifilar helical coil
   Material: MP35N nickel alloy
   Insulation: polyurethane
   Diameter of Shaft: 1.1 mm (3.5 FR)
   Maximum Insertion Diameter: 3.0 mm (9.0 FR)
   Length Option: 60 cm
   Splice Kit Available: no
   Lead Resistance: 50 ohms
   Other Special Characteristics:

6. **CONNECTOR**
   Type: pin with setscrew
   Interconnection to Other Manufacturers without Adapter: all 5-mm connectors (867—all 6-mm connectors)

   Adapter Available: yes
   Extension Kit Available: no
   New Connector Available: yes
   Conductor Material: 316L stainless steel
   Metals Compatible with Other Manufacturers' Connectors: yes
   Special Features:

PACESETTER SYSTEMS, INC.

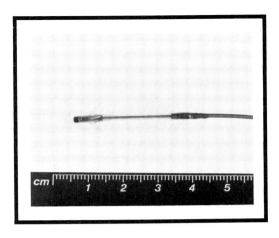
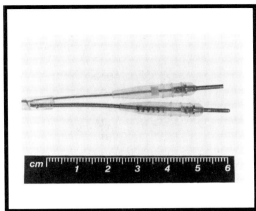

1. **IDENTIFICATION**
   Lead Model Number: 866
   Special Name:

2. **GENERAL DESCRIPTION**
   Intended Use: pervenous
   Designed for: right ventricle

3. **ELECTRODES**

	Electrode #1 (most distal)	Electrode #2 (next proximal)	Electrode #3 (next proximal)
Shape:	blunt ring	ring	
Surface Area:	8.0 mm²	48.0 mm²	
Material:	platinum-iridium	platinum-iridium	

   Remarks:

4. **FIXATION MECHANISM:**   tines

5. **WIRE**
   Configuration: coaxial helical coil (inner—trifilar, outer—quadrifilar)
   Material: MP35N nickel alloy
   Insulation: Silastic
   Diameter of Shaft: 1.5 mm (4.5 FR)
   Maximum Insertion Diameter: 3.0 mm (9.0 FR)
   Length Option: 60 cm
   Splice Kit Available: no
   Lead Resistance: 69 ohms each leg
   Other Special Characteristics:

6. **CONNECTOR**
   Type: bifurcated pin with setscrew
   Interconnection to Other Manufacturers without Adapter: 5-mm connectors

   Adapter Available: yes
   Extension Kit Available: no
   New Connector Available: no
   Conductor Material: 316L stainless steel
   Metals Compatible with Other Manufacturers' Connectors: yes
   Special Features:

PACESETTER SYSTEMS, INC.

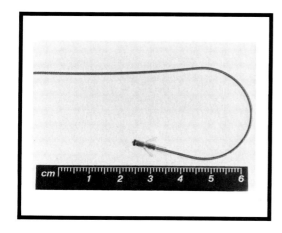
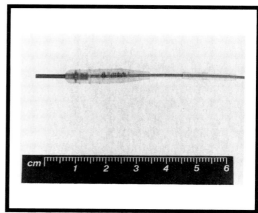

1. **IDENTIFICATION**
   Lead Model Number: 869
   Special Name:

2. **GENERAL DESCRIPTION**
   Intended Use: pervenous
   Designed for: right atrial appendage

3. **ELECTRODES**

	Electrode #1 (most distal)	Electrode #2 (next proximal)	Electrode #3 (next proximal)
Shape:	blunt ring		
Surface Area:	8.0 mm²		
Material:	platinum-iridium		

   Remarks:

4. **FIXATION MECHANISM:**   tines

5. **WIRE**
   Configuration: trifilar helical coil
   Material: MP35N nickel alloy
   Insulation: polyurethane
   Diameter of Shaft: 1.3 mm (3.8 FR)
   Maximum Insertion Diameter: 3.0 mm (9.0 FR)
   Length Option: 52 cm
   Splice Kit Available: no
   Lead Resistance: 330 ohms
   Other Special Characteristics: "J" curve for positional stability

6. **CONNECTOR**
   Type: pin with set screw
   Interconnection to Other Manufacturers without Adapter: all 5-mm connectors

   Adapter Available: yes
   Extension Kit Available: no
   New Connector Available: yes
   Conductor Material: 316L stainless steel
   Metals Compatible with Other Manufacturers' Connectors: yes
   Special Features:

SIEMENS-ELEMA

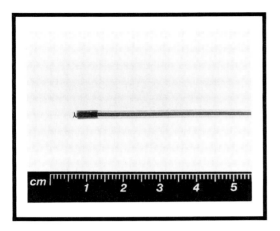 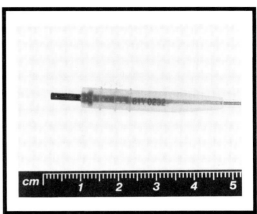

1. **IDENTIFICATION**
   Lead Model Number: 402S
   Special Name:

2. **GENERAL DESCRIPTION**
   Intended Use: pervenous
   Designed for: right atrium/right ventricle

3. **ELECTRODES**

	Electrode #1 (most distal)	Electrode #2 (next proximal)	Electrode #3 (next proximal)
Shape:	screw-helix		
Surface Area:	7 mm^2		
Material:	platinum		

   Remarks:

4. **FIXATION MECHANISM:**   screw-helix

5. **WIRE**
   Configuration: trifilar helical coil
   Material: MP35N nickel alloy
   Insulation: Silastic
   Diameter of Shaft: 2.2 mm (6.5 FR)
   Maximum Insertion Diameter: 2.7 mm (8.0 FR)
   Length Option: 60 cm
   Splice Kit Available: yes
   Lead Resistance: 85 ohms
   Other Special Characteristics:

6. **CONNECTOR**
   Type: pin with setscrew
   Interconnection to Other Manufacturers without Adapter: other 6-mm connectors

   Adapter Available: yes
   Extension Kit Available: yes
   New Connector Available: yes
   Conductor Material: stainless steel
   Metals Compatible with Other Manufacturers' Connectors: yes
   Special Features:

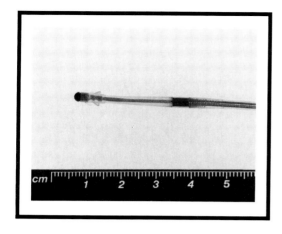
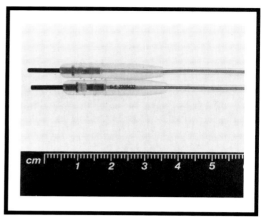

1. **IDENTIFICATION**
    Lead Model Number: 404B
    Special Name:

2. **GENERAL DESCRIPTION**
    Intended Use: pervenous
    Designed for: right ventricle

3. **ELECTRODES**

	Electrode #1 (most distal)	Electrode #2 (next proximal)	Electrode #3 (next proximal)
Shape:	hemispherical	ring	
Surface Area:	12 mm²	48 mm²	
Material:	vitreous carbon	platinum	

    Remarks: vitreous carbon has shown low and stable thresholds as well as reduced polarization losses

4. **FIXATION MECHANISM:**   tines

5. **WIRE**
    Configuration: trifilar helical coil
    Material: MP35N nickel alloy
    Insulation: Silastic
    Diameter of Shaft: 2.6 mm (8 FR)
    Maximum Insertion Diameter: 3.4 mm (11.0 FR)
    Length Option: 60 cm
    Splice Kit Available: no
    Lead Resistance: 85 ohms to tip, 60 ohms to ring
    Other Special Characteristics:

6. **CONNECTOR**
    Type: pin with setscrew
    Interconnection to Other Manufacturers without Adapter: other 5-mm connectors

    Adapter Available: yes
    Extension Kit Available: no
    Conductor Material: stainless steel
    Metals Compatible with Other Manufacturers' Connectors: yes
    Special Features:

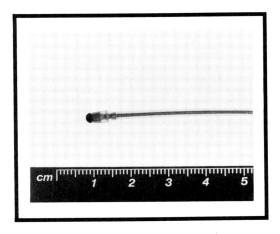 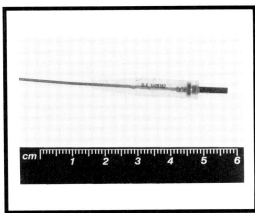

1. **IDENTIFICATION**
   Lead Model Number: 411S
   Special Name:

2. **GENERAL DESCRIPTION**
   Intended Use: pervenous
   Designed for: right ventricle

3. **ELECTRODES**

	Electrode #1 (most distal)	Electrode #2 (next proximal)	Electrode #3 (next proximal)
Shape:	hemispherical		
Surface Area:	12.0 mm^2		
Material:	vitreous carbon		

   Remarks: vitreous carbon has shown low and stable thresholds as well as reduced polarization losses

4. **FIXATION MECHANISM:**   flange

5. **WIRE**
   Configuration: bifilar helical coil
   Material: MP35N nickel alloy
   Insulation: Silastic
   Diameter of Shaft: 2.2 mm (6.5 FR)
   Maximum Insertion Diameter: 3.2 mm (10.0 FR)
   Length Option: 50 cm, 60 cm
   Splice Kit Available: yes
   Lead Resistance: 105 ohms (50 cm), 125 ohms (60 cm)
   Other Special Characteristics:

6. **CONNECTOR**
   Type: pin with setscrew
   Interconnection to Other Manufacturers without Adapter: other 6-mm connectors

   Adapter Available: yes
   Extension Kit Available: yes
   New Connector Available: yes
   Conductor Material: stainless steel
   Metals Compatible with Other Manufacturers' Connectors: yes
   Special Features:

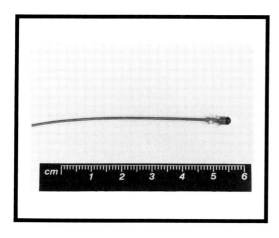
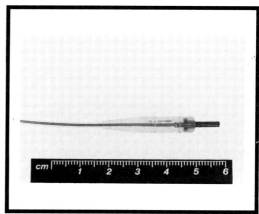

1. **IDENTIFICATION**
   Lead Model Number: 412S
   Special Name:

2. **GENERAL DESCRIPTION**
   Intended Use: pervenous
   Designed for: right atrium/right ventricle

3. **ELECTRODES**

	Electrode #1 (most distal)	Electrode #2 (next proximal)	Electrode #3 (next proximal)
Shape:	hemispherical		
Surface Area:	12 mm²		
Material:	vitreous carbon		

   Remarks: vitreous carbon has shown low and stable thresholds as well as reduced polarization losses

4. **FIXATION MECHANISM:**   tines

5. **WIRE**
   Configuration: bifilar helical coil
   Material: MP35N nickel alloy
   Insulation: Silastic
   Diameter of Shaft: 2.2 mm (6.5 FR)
   Maximum Insertion Diameter: 3.4 mm (11.0 FR)
   Length Option: 50, 60 cm
   Splice Kit Available: yes
   Lead Resistance: 105 ohms (50 cm), 125 ohms (60 cm)
   Other Special Characteristics:

6. **CONNECTOR**
   Type: pin with setscrew
   Interconnection to Other Manufacturers without Adapter: other 6-mm connectors

   Adapter Available: yes
   Extension Kit Available: yes
   New Connector Available: yes
   Conductor Material: stainless steel
   Metals Compatible with Other Manufacturers' Connectors: yes
   Special Features:

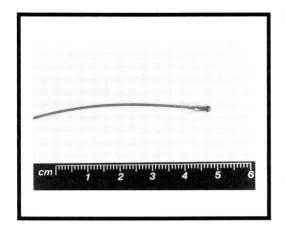
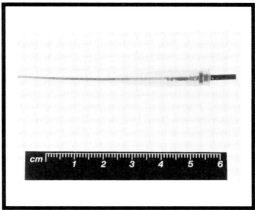

1. IDENTIFICATION
Lead Model Number: 415S
Special Name:

2. GENERAL DESCRIPTION
Intended Use: pervenous
Designed for: right atrium/right ventricle

3. ELECTRODES

	Electrode #1 (most distal)	Electrode #2 (next proximal)	Electrode #3 (next proximal)
Shape:	hemispherical		
Surface Area:	12.0 mm^2		
Material:	platinum		

Remarks:

4. FIXATION MECHANISM: tines

5. WIRE
Configuration: bifilar helical coil
Material: MP35N nickel alloy
Insulation: Silastic
Diameter of Shaft: 2.2 mm (6.5 FR)
Maximum Insertion Diameter: 3.4 mm (11.0 FR)
Length Option: 60 cm
Splice Kit Available: yes
Lead Resistance: 125 ohms
Other Special Characteristics:

6. CONNECTOR
Type: pin with setscrew
Interconnection to Other Manufacturers without Adapter: other 6-mm connectors

Adapter Available: yes
Extension Kit Available: yes
New Connector Available: yes
Conductor Material: stainless steel
Metals Compatible with Other Manufacturers' Connectors: yes
Special Features:

APPENDIX. ADDRESSES AND TELEPHONE NUMBERS OF MANUFACTURERS

DOMESTIC ADDRESSES

AMERICAN EDWARDS LABS
17221 Red Hills Avenue
P.O. Box 1150
Irvine, California 92714
Telephone: 800-424-3278

AMERICAN PACEMAKER CORP.
10 Sonar Drive
Woburn, Massachusetts 01801
Telephone: 617-890-5656

BIOTRONIK SALES
P.O. Box 1988
Lake Oswego, Oregon 97034
Telephone: 503-635-3594

CARDIAC CONTROL SYSTEMS, INC.
3 Commerce Boulevard
Palm Coast, Florida 32037
Telephone: 904-445-5450

CARDIAC PACEMAKERS, INC.
4100 North Hamlin Avenue
P.O. Box 43079
St. Paul, Minnesota 55164
Telephone: 612-638-4000

COOK PACEMAKER CORP.
P.O. Box 529
Leechburg, Pennsylvania 15656
Telephone: 412-845-8621

CORATOMIC, INC.
Box 434
Indiana, Pennsylvania 15701
Telephone: 412-349-1811

CORDIS CORP.
P.O. Box 025700
Miami, Florida 33102-5700
Telephone: 305-551-2000

DAIG CORP.
14901 Minnetonka Industrial Road
Minnetonka, Minnesota 55345
Telephone: 800-328-3873

INTERMEDICS, INC.
P.O. Box 617
240 Tarpon Inn Village
Freeport, Texas 77541
Telephone: 713-233-8611

MED TELECTRONICS LTD.
8515 East Orchard Road
Suite 208
Englewood, Colorado 80111
Telephone: 800-525-7001

MEDTRONIC INCORPORATED
6951 Central Avenue, N.E.
P.O. Box 1453
Minneapolis, Minnesota 55440
Telephone: 800-328-2518

PACESETTER SYSTEMS, INC.
12740 San Fernando Road
Sylmar, California 91342
Telephone: 213-362-6822

SIEMENS-ELEMA PACEMAKER DIVISION ELEMA-SCHONANDER, INC.
3260 North Palmer Drive
Shaumburg, Illinois 60195
Telephone: 312-397-5950

STIMULATION TECHNOLOGY, INC.
9440 Science Center Drive
Minneapolis, Minnesota 55428
Telephone: 612-535-0255

VITATRON MEDICAL
1 Gateway Center
Newton, Massachusetts 02158
Telephone: 617-964-1980

FOREIGN ADDRESSES

BIOTEC TECNOLOGIE BIOMEDICHE S.A.S.
Via Dell'Arcoveggio, 70
40129 Bologna, Italy
Telephone: 051-323186

CENTRO DE CONSTRUCCION DE
CARDIOESTIMUADORES DEL
URUGUAY
Casilla Postal P.O. Box 954
Montevideo, Uruguay
Telephone: 58-64-04

CARDIOFRANCE
Compagnie francaise
d'electrocardiologie
73, route de Neuilly-93160
Noisy-le-Grande, France

CORPOREL
Tour Roussel-Nobel-Cidex 3
92080 Paris La Defense
Telephone: 1-778-15-15

DEVICES IMPLANTS LTD.
(STIM-TECH)
4 Market Place
Herford SG14 IEB, England

ELA MEDICAL
100 rue Maurice Arnoux
92120 Montrouge, France
Telephone: 657 1151

ELEMA-SCHONANDER, INC
Siemens-Elema AB
517195 Solna, Sweden

LEM BIOMEDICA
50030 Cavallina di Mugelle
Firenze, Italy

MEDICAL DEVICES S.p.A.
Via del Crocifisso 39-Cap 50015
Ponte A Ema (Fi) Italy
Telephone: 055-643657-Telex 573156

SORIN MEDICA INTERNATIONAL
13040 Saluggio (Vercelli), Italy
28 rue Caroline, 92340
Bourg-la-Reine, France

TELECTRONICS
2 Sirius Road
Lane Grove
Box 333
P.O. Lane Cove
N.S.W. 2066 Australia

UNIVERSIDAD DE BUENOS AIRES
Facultad De Ingenieria
Paseo Colon 850
Buenos Aires, Argentina

VITATRON MEDICAL B.V.
P.O. Box 76
6950 AB Dieren
The Netherlands

INDEX

This index includes page numbers from both *A Guide to Cardiac Pacemakers* and this *Supplement*. *Italics* indicate a figure. A t indicates a table. A page number beginning with S indicates a page in the *Supplement*.

AGE
  implantation and, 2
  pacer dependency and, 9
  perforation and, 7
Air entrapment, pacemaker pouch and, 37, *40*
Air-fluid level, infection and, *64–65*, 68
Allen wrench, 2
American Pacemaker Corporation
  external pulse generators of, 446–447
  leads of, 352–355
  pacemakers of, 94–113
  programmers of *468*, 469, *470*, *471*
American Technology, Inc., pacemakers of, 114–115
Amperage, programming of, 22
ARCO-Intermedics, Inc., pacemakers of, 116–127
Arrhythmia
  iatrogenic, P-triggered ventricular pacemaker and, 78
  rate programming and, 16
ASVIP pacing, 5
Atrial pacing
  continuous asynchronous, *80*
  continuous sequential ventricular and, *79*
  P-inhibited, *80*
  P-triggered, *80*
  QRS-inhibited, 78, *79*, *80*
  sick sinus disease and, 2–3
  synchronous, 4–5
Atrial transport, VVI pacers and, 3
Atrioventricular conduction defects, 2–3
Atrioventricular pacing, 78, *79*, *81*
Automatic implantable cardioverter-defibrillator, S-5–S-6
Automatic interval, escape interval and, 74, *75*, *76*

BATTERY
  Catalyst Research Corporation, 86t–87t, *88*, *89*, *90*
  depletion of
    electrocardiographic evidence of, 71, 76
    output pulse and, 9

P-triggered ventricular pacemaker and, 78
  QRS-triggered mode and, 78
discharge projection of, *90*
expense and, 10
future developments in, 90
gas emission and, 40, 41, 83, 84
General Electric, 83
life expectancy of
  electrode size and, 2
  rate programming and, 16
  threshold programming and, 18
lithium
  advantages of, 10, 84
  follow-up of, 10–11
  identification of, 43, *43*, *44*, 85
  life expectancy of, 16–17
  radiology of, 43, *43*, *44*
  specifications of, 86t–87t
  types of, 84, 86t–87t
Mallory RM1, 83, 86t–87t
mercury-zinc
  degeneration of, 41–42, *42*
  disadvantages of, 10, 41
  fluoroscopy and, 41–42
  gas emission and, 40
  history of, 3, 10, 40, 83
  life expectancy of, 16–17
  specifications of, 86t–87t
  types of, 83
nickel cadmium
  history of, 1, 10, 83
  life expectancy of, 43, 83
  radiology of, *44*
  structure of, 43, *44*
nuclear
  disadvantages of, 10, 43–46
  history of, 1, 46
  structure of, *45*
  types of, 46
parameters of, 86t–87t
plutonium, *45*, 46, 83
promethium, 46, 83
rechargeable, 1, 10, 43, *44*, 83

Battery (*continued*)
    specifications of, 86t–87t
    tritium, 83
    types of, 10, 86t–87t. *See also* specific fuels
    Wilson Greatbatch, 84t, *85*, 86t–87t
    x-ray film of, *40, 42, 43, 44, 45, 89. See also*
        pacemaker atlas
Biotec-Tecnologie Biomediche, pacemakers
    of, 128–141
Biotronik
    external pulse generators of, 448, *S-26,*
        S-27, S-30, S-31
    leads of, 356–360, S-149–S-153
    monitor of, 514
    pacemakers of, 142–149, S-12–S-25
    pacing system analyzer of, 456
    programmers of, *472,* 473, *S-28,* S-29
    stimulator of, 507–508
Bisping leads, 5, *5*
Bradyarrhythmia, atrial, 33, *34*
Braided lead, 1
Butterfly, lead fracture and, *7*

CARBON, conduction and, 4
Carbon lead, 1, 4
Cardiac Control Systems, Inc.
    leads of, S-154–S-156
    pacemakers of, S-32–S-35
    programmer of, *S-36,* S-37
Cardiac failure, atrial synchronous pacing
    and, 4–5
Cardiac Pacemakers, Inc.
    leads of, 361–373, S-157
    pacemakers of, 150–159, S-38–S-45
    pacing system analyzer of, 457
    programmers of, *474,* 475, *476,* 477, S-46–S-
        51
CardioFrance, pacemakers of, 160–171
Cardiomyopathy, atrial synchronous pacing
    and, 4–5
Cardio-Pace Medical
    pacemakers of, S-52–S-53
    programmer of, S-55
Case, pacemaker, material of, 1
Catalyst Research Corporation batteries, 86t–
    87t, *88, 89, 90*
Catheter connection, pacer and, 7
Centro de Construcción de Cardioestimula-
    dores, pacemaker of, 172–173
Circuitry, pacemaker, 1
Clinic, pacemaker, 9–10
Code
    ICHD, 2, 2t, 3t
    radiographic identification, 527–531
Components, pacemaker, 1. *See also* Battery;
    Electrode; Lead
Conduction material, 4
Connector system, 1–2
    design of, S-135, *S-136*
    sizes of, S-143t–S-146t
Constant current pacemakers, 18–19

Cook Pacemaker Corporation, pacemakers of,
    174–179
Coratomic, Inc.
    leads of, 374–376
    pacemakers of, 180–193
Cordis Corporation
    connectors of, 2
    electrophysiology stimulator of, S-70–S-71
    external pulse generators of, 449–450, S-68–
        S-69
    leads of, 377–391, S-158–S-162
    pacemakers of, 194–211, S-56–S-67
    pacing system analyzer of, 458
    programmers of, *478,* 479, *480,* 481

DDD pacing, 5
Demand units, indications for, 4
Dependency, pacemaker, 9, 21–22
Diaphragmatic pacing, 6
Dislodgement, electrode
    fibrin sheath and, 30
    incidence of, 3
    radiology of, *50, 51, 52,* 53–56, *54, 55, 56*
Dressler's syndrome, myocardial perforation
    and, 60
Dual atrial and ventricular pacers, 5
DVI pacing, bifocal, 5

EDWARDS Pacemaker Systems, pacemakers of,
    212–215
Ela Medical
    monitor of, 515
    pacemakers of, 216–227, S-72–S-75
    pacing system analyzer of, 459
    programmer of, *482,* 483
Electrocardiogram
    atrioventricular sequential, P-inhibited
        atrial, P-triggered ventricular, QRS-
        inhibited ventricular, *81*
    continuous asynchronous ventricular
        mode, 71–74, *72, 73, 74, 75*
    electrode contact and, 74, *74*
    escape interval and, 20, 74, *75, 76, 79, 80*
    filing of, 22
    fusion beat on, *75, 76, 77, 78,* 78
    hysteresis and, 23
    implantation monitoring and, 8
    lead fracture on, 74
    magnet test and, 76, *76*
    myocardial perforation and, 57–60
    programming determination and, 21
    pseudofusion beat on, *75, 77, 78*
    P-triggered mode and, 78, *79*
    P-triggered QRS-inhibited ventricular
        mode, *81*
    QRS-inhibited sequential atrioventricular
        mode, 78, *79*
    QRS-inhibited ventricular mode and, 74–76,
        75, 76
    QRS-triggered ventricular mode and, 76–
        78, *77, 78*

R on T phenomenon on, 71, *73 77*
repetitive, reprogramming and, 80
Electrode
  bipolar, 1, 3
  coronary sinus and, 56–57, *58*
  design of, S-135–S-141, *S-137, S-138, S-139*
  dislocation of, 5, 37–38, *50, 51, 52, 53,* 56–57, *56. See also* Electrode, dislodgement of; Radiology, pacemaker failure and, electrode malposition in
  dislodgement of, *50, 51, 52,* 53–56, *54, 55, 56. See also* Electrode, dislocation of
  electromagnetic interference and, 3
  Elgiloy, 1, 32
  farfield potentials and, 3
  faulty contact of, electrocardiogram and, 74, *74*
  fixation of, 3–4, *4,* 5, *5, 6,* 27, *28,* 37–38
  flange-shaped, 37
  grasping, 37
  J-shaped, 5
  malposition of, radiology of, 30–31, *31, 32, 33, 34, 35, 36, 37,* 56–57, *56, 57, 58, 59. See also* Electrode, dislodgement of, radiology of
  material of, 1, 32–33
  placement of, correct, 1, 27, *28,* 29, *29*
  porous tip, *6, 443*
  position of, radiology of, 27–31, *28, 29, 30, 31, 32, 33, 34, 35, 36*
  screw-in, 3–4, *4, 5,* 27, *28*
  size of, 2, 18
  stability of, 3–4, *4,* 5, *5, 6,* 27, *28,* 37–38
  thrombus formation and, 37–38
  tined, 3, 37–38
  unipolar, 1, 3
  VVI pacers and, 3
Electromagnetic interference
  bipolar electrodes and, 3
  fixed rate discharge and, 74
  mode programming and, 20
  sensitivity and, 19, 23
Elgiloy electrode, 1, 32
Embolism, pulmonary, 43, 65
Epoxy silicone encapsulation, 40
Escape, false, 77, 78
Escape interval
  automatic interval and, 74, *75, 76, 79, 80*
  programming and, 20
Exit block, 49, *75*
External pacemaker, 3, 11, 445–454

FAILURE of pacemaker
  dependency and, 9
  detection of, 8, 9t
  dislodgement and, 5. *See also* Dislodgement, electrode
  inadequate connection and, 7
  monitoring and, 8, 9t
  perforation and, 6. *See also* Perforation
  pressure necrosis and, 7

radiology and. *See* Radiology, pacemaker failure and
  rate decay and, 18
  R-wave sensing and, 6–7
  sealing and, 7
  threshold increase and, 6
  wire fracture and, *7. See also* Lead, fracture of
Farfield potentials, bipolar electrodes and, 3
Fibrin sheath, 30
Fistula, bronchocutaneous, *67,* 68
Fixation, electode, 3–4, *4,* 5, *5, 6,* 27, *28,* 37–38
Fluid level, roentgenogram of, *64–65,* 68
Fluoroscopy
  implantation and, 32
  lead fracture and, 49
  mercury-zinc battery and, depletion of, 41–42, *42*
  myocardial perforation and, 60
  pacemaker identificaiton and, 42
Fracture
  lead. *See* Lead, fracture of
  pseudo-, 32, *39*
Fusion beat, *75, 76, 77,* 78, *78*

GAS formation, power source and, 40, 41, 83, 84
General Electric battery, 83
Greatbatch battery, 84t, *85,* 86t–87t

HEART block, 2
Helical coil lead, 1
History of pacemakers, 3–5
Hysteresis
  electrocardiogram and, 23
  programming of, 20, 23
  rate, 74, *76*

ICHD code, 2, 2t, 3t
Identification codes, radiographic, 527–531
Identification of pacemaker, 21, 42–43, 527–531
Impedance, lead, 4
Implantation
  epicardial, 27, *28*
  fluoroscopy and, 32
  pacemaker position and, 31
  radiology and. *See* Radiology, implantation and
  subclavian, *35*
  subxiphoid, 27, *28*
  thoracotomy and, 27, *29*
  transxiphoid, 27
Indications for pacing, 2–5
Infection, 3, *64–65,* 67–68, *67*
Infiltrate, lingular, *67*
Instromedix, Inc., monitor of, 451
Intermedics, Inc.
  external pulse generator of, 451
  leads of, 392–398, S-163–S-175

Intermedics, Inc. (*continued*)
  monitor of, 517
  pacemakers of, 228–239, S-76–S-87
  pacing system analyzer of, 460–462
  programmers of, *484*, 485, *486*, 487, *S-88*, S-89, *S-90*, S-91
Ionizing radiation, pacemaker function and, S-1–S-2
Iridium electrode, 1

J-SHAPED electrode, 5

KEITH spearpoint needle, *12*, 13

LEAD. *See also* Electrode
  bipolar, definition of, 1
  Bisping, 5, *5*
  braided, 1
  carbon, 1, 4
  connector system for, 1–2
  diameter of, 4
  durability of, 4
  fracture of
    causes of, 7
    configuration and, 33
    electrocardiographic evidence of, 74
    incidence of, 38, 49
    radiology of, 32, *38*, *39*, *46*, *47*, *48*, 49–50, *49*, *55*, *58*
    sites of, 49. *See also* Lead, fracture of, radiology of trauma and, *49*, 50
  impedance of, 4
  J-shaped, *34*
  material of, 1
  multifilar, 1
  Osypka, 4, *4*
  polyurethane, pseudofracture and, 32, *39*
  redundant, perforation and, 30, *31*
  resistance of, 1
  urethane insulation of, 4
LEM Biomedica, pacemakers of, 240–265
Life expectancy
  battery and
    lithium, 10, 16–17
    rate programming and, 16–17
  worst case programming and, 18
Lingula, infiltrate of, *67*
Lithium battery
  advantages of, 10, 84
  follow-up of, 10–11
  identification of, 43, *43*, *44*, 85
  life expectancy of, 16–17
  radiology of, 43, *43*, *44*
  specifications of, 86t–87t
  types of, 84, 86t–87t
Longevity of pacemaker. *See* Life expectancy

MAGNET
  effects of, 521–527
  Vitatron Medical, 504–505, *504, 505*

Magnet rate
  QRS-inhibited ventricular pacemaker and, 74, 76, *76*
  QRS-triggered mode and, 78
Magnetic resonance, pacemaker function and, S-2
Mallory RM1 battery, 83
Manufacturers, addresses of, 533–534, S-199–S-200
Marquette ECG machine, 9
Medcor, pacemakers of, 266–273
Mediastinoscope, electrode insertion with, 4
Medtronic, Inc.
  connectors of, 2
  external pulse generator of, 452, *S-108*, S-109, *S-112*, S-113, *S-114*, S-115
  leads of, 399–419, S-176–S-184
  monitor of, 518
  pacemakers of, 274–293, S-92–S-105
  pacing system analyzers of, 463–464, S-106–S-107
  programmers of, *488*, 489, *490*, 491, *492*, 493, *494*, 495, *S-116*, S-117
  stimulator of, 509–511, *S-110*, S-111
Mercury-zinc battery
  degeneration of, 41–42, *42*
  disadvantages of, 10, 41
  fluoroscopy and, 41–42
  gas emission and, 40
  history of, 3, 10, 40, 83
  life expectancy of, 16–17
  radiology of, *40*, *42*
  specifications of, 86t–87t
  structure of, 41, *41*
  types of, 83
Mode
  atrioventricular sequential, P-inhibited atrial, P-triggered ventricular, QRS-inhibited ventricular, *81*
  code, 2, 2t, 3t. *See also* ICHD code
  continuous asynchronous ventricular, 71–74, *72*, *73*, *74*, *75*
  programming of, 20. *See also* specific modes
  P-triggered, QRS-inhibited ventricular, *81*
  P-triggered ventricular, 78, *79*
  QRS-inhibited sequential atrioventricular, 78, *79*
  QRS-inhibited ventricular, 74–76, *75*, *76*
  QRS-triggered ventricular, 76–78, *77*, *78*
  R-wave triggered, 20
Monitoring
  pacemaker failure and, 8, 9t
  telephone, 10–11
Multistrand lead, 1

NECROSIS, pressure, 7
Nickel alloy electrode, 1
Nickel cadmium battery
  history of, 1, 10, 83
  life expectancy of, 43, 83

radiology of, *44*
structure of, 43, *44*
Noncapture, ventricular, *73*, 74
Nuclear battery
  disadvantages of, 10, 43–46, 83
  history of, 1, 46, 83
  structure of, *45*
  types of, 46, 83
Nuclear pacemaker, identification of, 532

OSYPKA leads, dislodgement of, 4, *4*

PACEMAKER syndrome, atrial synchronous pacing and, 5
Pacesetter Systems, Inc.
  external pulse generator of, 453
  leads of, 420–427, S-185–S-192
  pacemakers of, 294–299, S-118–S-127
  programmer of, *496, 497*
Palpitations, demand units and, 4
Pencil magnet, programming and, *11*
Perforation, myocardial
  diagnosis of, 57–60,m *60, 61*
  electrocardiogram and, 57–60
  incidence of, 38
  pacemaker failure and, 6, 7
  radiology and, 30, *31, 36*, 60, *60, 61*
  time of, 32
  ultrasound and, *36*
Physiologic pacing, 5
Platinum electrode, 1
Plutonium battery, 1, *45*, 46, 83
Position, implant
  cephalic vein as, 3
  monitoring, 8
  subclavian vein as, 3
Position code, 2t, 3t
Postcardiotomy syndrome, myocardial perforation and, 60
Potentials, skeletal muscle, sensitivity and, 19
Pouch, pacer, 7
Power source. *See* Battery
Powers Medical Systems, Inc., monitor of, 519
Pressure necrosis, pacer failure and, 7
Programming
  amperage, 17–18. *See also* Programming, output
  devices for, 467
  escape interval, 20
  hysteresis, 20
  mode, 20
  output
    advantages of, 6, 16
    magnet and, 14–15
  manufacturers with, 6t
  on/off time and, 19
  parameters of, 18–19
  pulse width and, 19
  strength-duration curve and, 19
  technique of, 22

threshold problems and, 6, 17
parameters of, 7t, 17–20
pulse width, 13–14, *13*
rate
  advantages of, 16, 18
  arrhythmia and, 16
  battery life and, 16
  cardiac output and, 16
  General Electric, 11, *11*
  history of, 11–14, *11, 12, 13*, 17–18
  magnet and
    effects of, 521–527
    history of, 15
    pencil, *11*
    rotating, 13–14, *13*
  parameters of, 18
  sinus rhythm and, 16, 18
  spearpoint needle and, *12*, 13
refractory period, 20
sensitivity, 19
techniques of
  amperage in, 22
  hysteresis in, 23
  information on, 21
  initiation of, 21
  output and, 22
  pacemaker dependency and, 21–22
  pacemaker identification and, 20–21
  prerequisites of, 20–21
  pulse width in, 22
  record-keeping and, 23
  refractory period setting in, 23
  safety in, 21–22
  sensitivity and, 23
  sinus rhythm in, 21
  telemetry and, 21
  voltage in, 22
  threshold problems and, 6, 17
Promethium battery, 46, 83
Pseudofusion beat, *75, 77*, 78
Pulse voltage, magnet control of, 15
Pulse width, programming of, 13–14, *13*, 19, 22

R on T phenomenon, 71, *73, 77*
R wave
  mode programming and, 20
  monitoring, 8
  recognition of, failure of, 19
  sensitivity setting and, 23
R-wave inhibited (VVI) pacer, 2
R-wave sensitivity, 6–7
Radiofrequency pacer, 14, *15, 16*
Radiology
  automatic implantable cardioverter-defibrillator and, S-5–S-6
  battery and, depletion of, 41–42, *42*
    lithium, 43
    mercury-zinc, 40, 41–42, *42*
    type of, *85, 89*. *See also* pacemaker atlas

Radiology (*continued*)
  bronchocutaneous fistula and, *67*, 68
  electrode dislodgement and, *50, 51, 52,* 53–56, *54, 55, 56*
  fluid level and, *64–65,* 68
  implantation and, S-2–S-3, *S-4*
    atrial, 31, *33, 34*
    cephalic approach and, 29, *29*
    epicardial, 27, *28*
    jugular approach and 29, *29*
    lead in, length of, 30, *31*
    malposition and, 30–31, *31, 32, 33, 34, 35, 36, 37*
    screw-in electrodes and, 27, *28*
    sinus, 30–31, *32*
    subclavian approach and, 29
  lead and
    extraction of, S-3, *S-5*
    fracture of, 32, *38, 39*
    J-shaped, *34*
    pseudofracture of, 32, *39*
    redundant, 30, *31*
  pacemaker failure and
    electrode dislodgement in, *50, 51, 52,* 53–56, *54, 55, 56. See also* Radiology, pacemaker failure and, electrode malposition in
    electrode malposition in, 56–57, *56, 57, 58, 59. See also* Radiology, pacemaker failure and, dislodgement in
    exit block in, 49
    infection in, *64–65,* 67–68, *67*
    lead fracture in, 49–50, *38, 39, 46, 47, 48, 49, 55, 58*
    myocardial perforation in, 60, *60, 61*
    pulmonary embolism in, 65
    thrombosis in, *62–63,* 65
  pacemaker identification and, 42–43
  twiddler's syndrome and, *52,* 53–56, *53, 55*
Rechargeable pacemaker, 1, 3, 10, 43, *44,* 83
Record-keeping, programming and, 23
Redundant pacer systems, 9
Refractory period
  programming of, 20, 23
  QRS-inhibited ventricular pacemaker and, 74
  QRS-triggered ventricular pacemaker and, 76–77
Runaway pacemaker, 71, *73*

SEALING, hermetic, power source and, 10
Sensitivity
  programming of, 19, 23
  R-wave, 6–7
Sick sinus disease, 2–3, 31
Siemens-Elema
  leads of, S-193–S-197
  pacemakers of, 300–315, S-128–S-131
  programmers of, *498, 499, 500,* 501
Silver alloy, conduction and, 4

Sinus, coronary, electrode malposition in, 30–31, *32, 35,* 56–57, *58*
Sinus node disorders, 2, 3
Sinus rhythm, normal, rate programming and, 16, 17, 18, 21
Size, pacemaker, 8t, 10
Sleeve, lead fracture and, 7
Spearpoint needle, programming and, *12,* 13
Staphylococcus aureus, 67
Strength-duration curve, output programming and, 19, 22
Streptococcus epidermis, 68
Superior vena cava syndrome, *62–63,* 65

TAMPONADE, cardiac, myocardial perforation and, 60
Telectronics
  leads of, 428–436
  pacemakers of, 316–337
  pacing system analyzer of, 465
  programmer of, *502,* 503
Telemetry
  initiation of programming and, 21
  multiple, 17
Telephone monitoring, 8, 9t, 10–11
Thoracotomy, 27, 29, 60
Threshold
  changes in, 8
  control of, 14, 18–19
  electrode malposition and, 53
  exit block and, 49
  high, 6, 16, 74, *75*
  low, monitoring, *8*
  Osypka leads and, 4
  programming of, 14, 18–19
Thrombosis, 37–38, *62–63,* 65
"Thru-and-thru" hole, 7
Transvenous approach, 3
Trauma, lead fracture and, *49,* 50
Tricuspid valve malfunction, 67
Tritium battery, 83
Twiddler's syndrome, *52,* 53–56, *53, 55*

ULTRASOUND, catheter position and, 32, *36–37*
Urethane insulation, leads and, 4

VALVE malfunction, 67
Vario function, 8
VAT pacing, 4–5
VATP pacing, 5
Ventricular pacing
  continuous asynchronous, 71–74, *72, 73, 74, 75*
  continuous sequential atrial and, *79*
  P-triggered, 78, *79*
  P-triggered, QRS-inhibited, *81*
  QRS-inhibited, 74–76, *75, 76, 77*
  QRS-inhibited sequential atrial and, 78, *79*
  QRS-triggered, 76–78, *77, 78*

Vitatron Medical
  external pulse generator of, 454
  leads of, 437–439
  magnet (programmer) of, 504–505, *504, 505*
  monitor of, 520
  pacemakers of, 338, 347, S-132–S-133
  pacing system analyzer of, 466
  programmer (magnet) of, 504–505, *504, 505*

Voltage, programming of, 22
Voltage doubler, 19
VVI pacer, 2

Wave filters, 3
Waveform analysis, definition of, 9
Wilson Greatbatch batteries, 84t, *85*, 86t–87t